AMERICAN DIETETIC ASSOCIATION

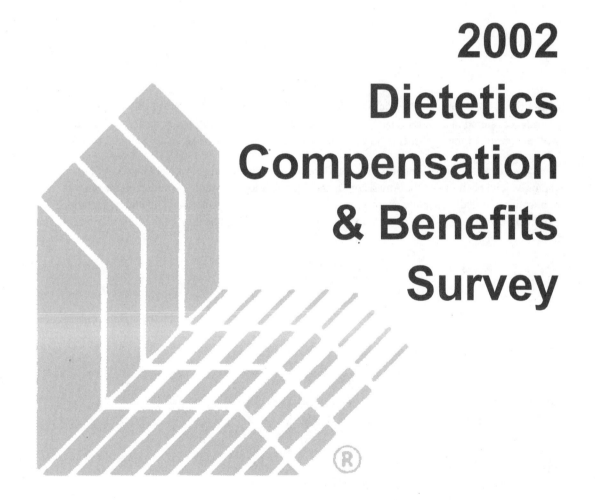

2002
Dietetics
Compensation
& Benefits
Survey

10 9 8 7 6 5 4 3 2 1

Library of Congress Cataloging-in-Publication Data

American Dietetic Association.
  2002 dietetics compensation & benefits survey / American Dietetic
Association.
     p. cm.
  ISBN 0-88091-316-9
  1. Dietitians--Salaries, etc.--United States. I. Title.

RM218.5 .A446 2003
331.2'81'6132--dc21
                                    2002152590

Preface

Over the years, the American Dietetic Association (ADA) has received many requests from members for objective, reliable information about industry norms for pay and benefit levels for the dietetics profession. Database surveys have been periodically conducted, providing generalized salary information for the major dietetics practice areas. However, many members wanted more specific information, and the concept of a salary survey by specific job title was suggested to ADA Chief Executive Officer Ronald Moen at the Association's Food and Nutrition Conference and Exhibition in St. Louis, Missouri, in October 2001. The ADA formed a Salary Survey Work Group shortly thereafter, with the Group's work culminating in the ADA's first Compensation and Benefits Survey, mailed in Summer 2002. This publication is a detailed report of the findings from that survey, which was conducted to provide an authoritative source of data on salaries, benefits, and work settings for core jobs in dietetics.

Since the ADA had never before conducted a compensation and benefits survey, the Association did not have on file position descriptions that could be used to formulate lists of job titles and descriptors, critical elements in such a survey. Therefore, the ADA issued a "call for job descriptions" in early 2002. The response from ADA members was very positive, and nearly 500 job descriptions were received. The ADA augmented these descriptions through interviews with employers and dietetics professionals in various practice areas and selected some fifty positions believed to account for over 80% of all dietetics employment. These are the core positions used for the survey instrument. Full descriptions are included in the companion publication, *Job Descriptions: Models for the Dietetics Profession.*

Current plans are for this survey to be conducted on a biennial basis. This authoritative source of data on salaries, benefits, and work settings will be an asset to professionals and their employers in all major dietetics practice settings, in addition to providing reference material for self-employed dietetics professionals.

Acknowledgments

The American Dietetic Association wishes to thank the nearly 500 members who shared their job descriptions, the members who provided valuable feedback throughout the development process, and the more than 13,000 ADA members and dietetics professionals who responded to the salary survey. Additional thanks go to Betsy A. Hornick, MS, RD, who worked in a consultant capacity to help develop the job titles and descriptors that were fundamental to this process.

Ronald S. Moen
Chief Executive Officer

Barbara J. Visocan, MS, RD, LD, FADA
Vice President, Member Services
Chair, Salary Survey Work Group

SALARY SURVEY WORK GROUP

Joe Bryk, PhD, Director, Association Research

Lorri Fishman, MS, RD, LD, formerly Project Manager, Knowledge Center

Jim Fitzpatrick, Vice President, Marketing and Communications

Karri Looby, MS, RD, LD, Director, Membership Marketing and Governance

Pam Michael, MBA, RD, LD, Director, Health Care Financing

Lori Porter, RD, LD, Director, Practice

Contents

TABLES

3. RD Compensation

4. RD Salary Calculation Worksheet

TABLES

5. DTR Compensation

6. DTR Salary Calculation Worksheet

TABLES

7. **Compensation By Position**
    broken out by years in field, years in position, education, credentials held, employer status, and responsibilities

TABLES

7. Compensation By Position (continued)
broken out by years in field, years in position, education, credentials held, employer status, and responsibilities

TABLES

8. Benefits

TABLES

10. Appendix

1. Executive Summary

Responding to member requests, the American Dietetic Association (ADA) has completed its first comprehensive survey of compensation and benefits in the dietetics profession.

Methodology

The survey was conducted across a probability sample drawn from the population of all domestic Active ADA members (N = 55,084) plus all domestic nonmembers (N = 18,654) maintaining current registration as a Registered Dietitian (RD) or Dietetic Technician, Registered (DTR). To preserve confidentiality of response, an outside research company was contracted to collect data via mail survey, which was conducted July 10 through August 26, 2002.

The survey breaks new ground in presenting results not only at the level of registration (RD, DTR) or in the context of various practice areas, but also in terms of the specific jobs (including nontraditional jobs) dietetics professionals hold. A key question asked respondents to identify the one position (from a recently developed set of 58 core positions) that most closely matched their actual employment. Compensation data are thus now available for the specific jobs that account for an estimated 95% of dietetics employment.

From the mailed sample of 30,000, a total of 13,694 usable responses was received — a 46% response rate. The strong response rate, plus the fact that nearly one in five professionals is represented in the tabulated sample, makes this the most exhaustive investigation to date of compensation in the dietetics profession.

Dietetics Employment

Slightly more than one in five dietetics professionals (21%) reported they are not currently employed or self-employed in a dietetics-related position. Survey results reflect the 10,829 sample members who indicated they are currently employed in the profession.

Practitioner Profile

97% of practitioners are female. Median age is 43 years; 11% are 55 or older, and 27% are under 35. 3% indicate they are of Hispanic heritage; 8% indicate a race other than white.

Virtually all RDs hold at least a bachelor's degree, with 45% holding master's degrees and 3% doctoral degrees. Among DTRs, 26% hold a bachelor's degree or higher.

85% of RDs are members of the ADA; in contrast, only 55% of responding DTRs are members. 51% of RDs and 6% of DTRs reported holding a state license (not required in all states). 16% of RDs and 6% of DTRs hold one or more specialty certifications (e.g., CNSD, CDE, FADA, CSR).

The typical (median) practitioner has 15 years of work experience in dietetics/nutrition (excluding time taken off to return to school, raise a family, or work in other areas).

Employers

10% of practitioners are self-employed (primarily RDs); 30% work for a for-profit firm, 40% for a nonprofit, and 19% for the government.

The most common employment setting for both RDs and DTRs was a hospital (33% and 37%, respectively). 32% of DTRs work in an extended-care facility, compared to only 10% of RDs. 10% of RDs work in a clinic or ambulatory care center, compared to only 2% of DTRs. 9% of both groups work in a community or public health program. Practitioners also reported employment in a wide variety of other settings.

Positions Held

Based on their selection of one most closely matching core position, dietetics professionals are employed or self-employed across a variety of primary practice areas:

Practice Area	RDs	DTRs
clinical nutrition — acute care/inpatient	28%	41%
clinical nutrition — ambulatory care	14%	1%
clinical nutrition — long term care	12%	20%
community	11%	10%
food and nutrition management	13%	20%
consultation and business	11%	2%
education and research	6%	1%

Among RDs, the positions most commonly held included Clinical Dietitian (16%); Outpatient Dietitian, General (4%); Outpatient Dietitian, Specialist — Diabetes (4%); Clinical Dietitian, Long-Term Care (12%); WIC Nutritionist (5%); Director of Food and Nutrition Services (5%); and Clinical Nutrition Manager (4%).

Among DTRs, the positions most commonly held included Dietetic Technician, Clinical (39%); Dietetic Technician, Long-Term Care (16%); WIC Nutritionist (7%); Director of Food and Nutrition Services (6%); and Dietetic Technician, Foodservice Management (10%).

Position Characteristics

6% of RDs and 2% of DTRs indicated they are owners or partners in their practice, while 2% of RDs and less than 1% of DTRs reported an executive level of responsibility. 22% of all practitioners are directors or managers, and 21% are supervisors or coordinators (results are similar for RDs and DTRs).

48% of RDs and 51% of DTRs reported they directly or indirectly supervise employees; 27% of RDs and 24% of DTRs reported managing a budget.

The typical (median) practitioner has been in the reported position for 5 years, with 31% in the job for less than 3 years and 33% in the job for 10 years or more.

RD Compensation

68% of practicing RDs reported working in their primary dietetics-related position full time (defined as at least 35 hours per week for at least 48 weeks per year). Because the prevalence of part-time employment can make salary comparisons difficult, compensation is reported in two ways: in terms of *hourly wage,* and in terms of *total cash compensation* (which includes not only salary but also earnings from bonuses, commissions, profit sharing, etc. — frequently important compensation components for consultants, executives, and those in sales positions). Hourly wage is assessed for all respondents; total cash compensation is examined only for those working full time for at least 1 year in the position.

Among all RDs in all positions, the median hourly wage as of April 1, 2002, was $22.00 per hour. If annualized (× 40 hours/week × 52 weeks/year), this equates to a salary of $45,760 per year. Median total cash compensation for RDs employed in the position full time for at least 1 year was $45,800.

These results are significantly higher than the most current Dietitian and Nutritionist wage estimates published by the Bureau of Labor Statistics, and the most recently published data from the ADA member database. However, survey estimates are significantly more current than either of those sources, and reflect a somewhat different population than either.

Of interest is the range of RD compensation:

All RDs	Hourly Wage	Total Cash
10th percentile (10% earn less)	$16.20	$34,000
25th percentile (25% earn less)	$18.75	$38,900
50th percentile (50% earn less)	$22.00	$45,800
75th percentile (75% earn less)	$26.79	$56,000
90th percentile (90% earn less)	$33.65	$72,000

Factors showing the strongest association with compensation levels for RDs include number of years of experience, level of supervisory responsibility, budget responsibility, and practice area: clinical and community positions tend to pay less, whereas consultation and business positions pay more.

The highest-paying non-academic positions held primarily by RDs include:

	Median Hourly Wage	Median Total Cash
Executive-level Professional	$34.86	$77,000
Research & Development Nutritionist	$30.30	$64,400
Public Relations or Marketing Professional	$29.43	$62,500
Director of Nutrition	$29.23	$67,500
School/Child Care Nutritionist	$26.44	$52,900
Sales Representative	$25.96	$70,000
Consultant — Communications	$25.73	$52,500
Director of Food and Nutrition Services	$25.07	$53,000
Clinical Nutrition Manager	$25.00	$51,900
Consultant — Community and/or Corporate Programs	$25.00	$47,100

DTR Compensation

75% of DTRs reported working in their primary dietetics-related position full time (at least 35 hours per week, at least 48 weeks per year).

Among all DTRs in all positions, the median hourly wage as of April 1, 2002, was $14.74 per hour; if annualized, this equals a salary of $30,660 per year. Median total cash compensation for DTRs employed in the position full time for at least 1 year was $31,000.

As with RDs, these current survey estimates are higher than those most recently published by BLS or ADA, but similar factors account for the discrepancies.

DTR compensation also spans a considerable range:

All DTRs	Hourly Wage	Total Cash
10th percentile (10% earn less)	$11.31	$23,900
25th percentile (25% earn less)	$12.82	$27,000
50th percentile (50% earn less)	$14.74	$31,000
75th percentile (75% earn less)	$16.97	$36,300
90th percentile (90% earn less)	$20.19	$43,100

Factors showing the strongest association with compensation levels for DTRs include number of years of experience, budget responsibility, size of organization, and practice area (on average, clinical and community positions receive lower compensation than others).

The highest-paying positions held by substantial numbers of DTRs include:

	Median Hourly Wage	Median Total Cash
Director of Food and Nutrition Services	$18.03	$40,000
Clinical Dietitian, Long Term Care	$15.39	$32,000
Dietetic Technician, Foodservice Management	$15.38	$32,900

Benefits

Although a significant fraction of them are employed part time, dietetics practitioners as a whole enjoy considerable fringe benefits from their work:

All Practitioners	% offered
paid vacation, personal time off	81%
paid holidays	75%
paid sick days	74%
medical insurance, group plan or savings account	81%
dental insurance or group plan	73%
prescription drug benefit	68%
vision insurance or group plan	54%
life insurance	70%
disability insurance (long- and/or short-term)	61%
defined contribution retirement plan	63%
defined benefit retirement plan (pension)	45%
stock options, ESOP	9%
profit sharing	8%
funding for professional development	59%
professional society dues	22%
college tuition assistance	42%
employee assistance or wellness program	41%
comp time or flex time	35%
fitness benefit	29%
extended and/or paid parental leave	26%
on-site child care or allowance	12%
telecommuting	7%

In many instances these percentages compare favorably with a reference group of professional/ technical employees in private industry (BLS data).

Future Surveys

Current plans are for this survey to be conducted on a biennial basis. This authoritative source of data on salaries, benefits and work settings should prove to be an asset to professionals and their employers in all major dietetics practice settings, as well as providing reference material for self-employed dietetics professionals.

2. Findings

Over the years, the American Dietetic Association (ADA) has received many requests from members for objective, reliable information about industry norms on pay and benefit levels for the dietetics profession. Database surveys have been periodically conducted, providing generalized salary information for the major dietetics practice areas. However, many members wanted more specific information and suggested the concept of a salary survey by specific job title. This document reports the results of the first such comprehensive survey of compensation and benefits in the dietetics profession.

This *Findings* section provides an overview of survey results: describing the research methodology, profiling survey respondents, and discussing compensation and benefits from a variety of perspectives. Detailed tables follow, showing how compensation for Registered Dietitians (RDs) and Dietetic Technicians, Registered (DTRs) is influenced by a variety of factors. Similar tables show compensation for nearly 50 distinct dietetics-related jobs. The report also features two easy-to-use Salary Calculation Worksheets (one for RDs, one for DTRs), which make exploration of compensation in a variety of employment situations possible. The report concludes with tables detailing benefits offered in dietetics-related employment, and further tables describing practitioners and their employment situations.

Methodology

The survey was conducted across a probability sample drawn from the population of all domestic Active ADA members (N = 55,084) plus all domestic nonmembers (N = 18,654) maintaining current registration as an RD or DTR. To preserve confidentiality of response, an outside research firm was contracted to collect data via mail survey, which was conducted July 10 through August 26, 2002.

The survey breaks new ground in presenting results not only at the level of registration (RD, DTR) or in the context of various practice areas, but also in terms of the specific jobs (including nontraditional jobs) dietetics professionals hold. A key question asked respondents to identify the one position (from a recently developed set of 58 core positions) that most closely matched their actual employment. Compensation data are thus now available for the specific jobs that account for an estimated 95% of dietetics employment.

From the mailed sample of 30,000, a total of 13,694 usable responses was received — a 46% response rate. The margin of error for all practitioners is ±0.9%; for practicing RDs, ±0.9%; for practicing DTRs, ±2.1%. The strong response rate, plus the fact that nearly one in five professionals is represented in the tabulated sample, makes this the most exhaustive investigation to date of compensation in the dietetics profession.

Dietetics Employment

The survey sought to measure compensation for dietetics-related employment, which was purposely conceived broadly:

> A dietetics-related position is considered to be any position that requires or makes use of your education, training, and/or experience in dietetics or nutrition, including situations outside of "traditional" dietetics practice.

By way of example, respondents were referred to an enclosure naming and briefly describing 58 core dietetics positions (see "Position Descriptions," page 173 in the *Appendix*). These positions included not only "traditional" dietetics jobs such as Clinical Dietitian, Outpatient Dietitian, or WIC Nutritionist, but also jobs in such areas as consulting, sales, and communications.

Based on this definition of dietetics-related employment, slightly more than one in five dietetics professionals (21%) reported they are not currently employed or self-employed in a dietetics-related position. This is disproportionately true for the small group of professionals not currently registered as RDs or DTRs.

Exhibit 2.1

Incidence of Dietetics-Related Employment

	# responding	% in dietetics
RDs	11,607	79%
DTRs	1,892	79%
non-registered practitioners	195	57%
all practitioners	13,694	79%

The balance of the results discussed reflect the 10,829 sample members who indicated they are currently employed or self-employed in a dietetics-related position ("practitioners"). Those who were employed or self-employed in more than one such position were asked to respond only for what they considered to be their *primary* dietetics-related position.

Practitioner Profile

97% of practitioners are female. The median age is 43; 11% are 55 or older, and 27% are under 35. 3% indicated Hispanic heritage; 8% indicated a race other than white.

Exhibit 2.2

Age (years)

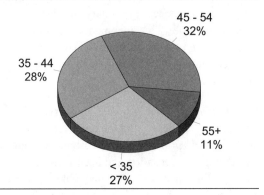

base: 10,829 practitioners

Virtually all RDs hold at least a bachelor's degree, with 45% holding master's degrees and 3% doctoral degrees. Among DTRs, 26% hold a bachelor's degree or higher.

Exhibit 2.3

Education (Highest Degree Attained)

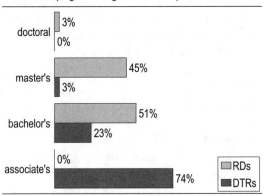

base: 9,220 practicing RDs; 1,498 practicing DTRs

85% of practicing RDs are members of the ADA, compared to only 55% of practicing DTRs. 51% of RDs and 6% of DTRs reported holding a state license (not required in all states). 16% of RDs and 6% of DTRs hold one or more specialty certifications (for example, CNSD, CDE, FADA, CSR, CSP, CHE, CDM, CFPP, CFE, CFM).

Exhibit 2.4

Credentials

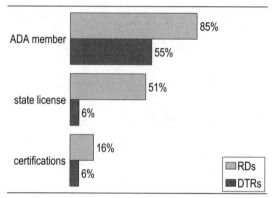

base: 9,220 practicing RDs; 1,498 practicing DTRs

The typical (median) RD reports 15 years of work experience in dietetics/nutrition (excluding time taken off to return to school, raise a family, or work in other areas); the median for DTRs was slightly lower (12 years). 35% of all practitioners have 20 or more years of work experience in dietetics/nutrition, whereas 19% have less than 5 years. Median year of initial registration was 1988 for RDs and 1994 for DTRs.

Exhibit 2.5

Years in Field

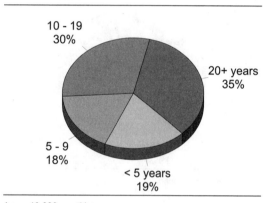

base: 10,829 practitioners

Employers

10% of practitioners are self-employed, 30% work for a for-profit firm, 40% for a nonprofit, and 19% for government. Self-employment is more common among RDs than DTRs (11% versus 2%, respectively), while a greater proportion of DTRs are found in nonprofit settings (38% of RDs, 48% of DTRs).

Exhibit 2.6

Employer Status

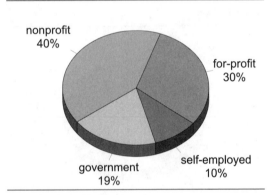

base: 10,829 practitioners

The most common employment setting for both RDs and DTRs is a hospital (33% and 37%, respectively). 32% of DTRs work in an extended care facility, compared to only 10% of RDs. 10% of RDs work in a clinic or ambulatory care center, compared to only 2% of DTRs. 9% of both groups work in a community or public health program.

Exhibit 2.7

Work Setting

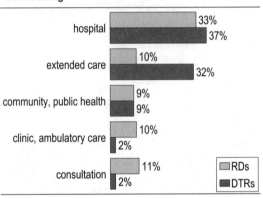

base: 9,220 practicing RDs; 1,498 practicing DTRs

11% of RDs work private practice/consultation to individuals or consultation/contract services to organizations, compared to only 2% of DTRs. Other settings in which at least 2% of practitioners are employed include college or university faculties, government agencies, school food service, contract food management companies, food manufacturers/distributors/retailers, and managed care organizations/physicians/other healthcare providers.

The typical practitioner works in an organization employing 534 people at all locations, with RDs tending to work in larger organizations than DTRs (medians 603 and 354, respectively).

Exhibit 2.8

Size of Organization

Number of Employees, All Locations

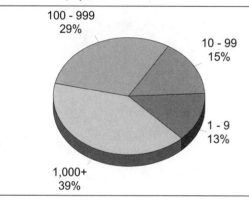

100 - 999 29%

10 - 99 15%

1 - 9 13%

1,000+ 39%

base: 10,829 practitioners

Positions Held

Respondents were asked to review a list of 58 core position titles and brief descriptions and identify the one description that most closely matched their primary position, even if the job title differed from their own (see page 173 in *Appendix* for the full set of position descriptions).

95% of responding practitioners found a match; thus the compensation data reported here represents the vast majority of dietetics employment situations.

The 58 positions were grouped into seven distinct practice areas, with acute care/inpatient the most prevalent, and education/research the least:

Exhibit 2.9

Practice Area, Primary Position

	RDs	DTRs
clinical nutrition — acute care/inpatient	28%	41%
clinical nutrition — ambulatory care	14%	1%
clinical nutrition — long term care	12%	20%
community	11%	10%
food and nutrition management	13%	20%
consultation and business	11%	2%
education and research	6%	1%

base: 9,220 practicing RDs; 1,498 practicing DTRs

Among RDs, the most commonly held positions included:

Exhibit 2.10

Highest Incidence Positions — RDs

	RDs
Clinical Dietitian	16%
Clinical Dietitian, Specialist — Renal	3%
Outpatient Dietitian, General	4%
Outpatient Dietitian, Specialist — Diabetes	4%
Outpatient Dietitian, Specialist — Renal	3%
Clinical Dietitian, Long Term Care	12%
WIC Nutritionist	5%
Public Health Nutritionist	3%
Director of Food and Nutrition Services	5%
Clinical Nutrition Manager	4%
Private Practice Dietitian — Patient/Client Nutrition Care	3%

base: 9,220 practicing RDs

Among DTRs, the most common positions were:

Exhibit 2.11

Highest Incidence Positions — DTRs

	DTRs
Dietetic Technician, Clinical	39%
Clinical Dietitian, Long Term Care	4%
Dietetic Technician, Long Term Care	16%
WIC Nutritionist	7%
Director of Food and Nutrition Services	6%
Dietetic Technician, Foodservice Management	10%

base: 1,498 practicing DTRs

Position Characteristics

6% of RDs and 2% of DTRs indicated they are owners of or partners in their practice, while 2% of RDs and less than 1% of DTRs reported an executive level of responsibility. 22% of practitioners overall are directors or managers, and 21% are supervisors or coordinators (results similar between RDs and DTRs).

Exhibit 2.12

Responsibility Level

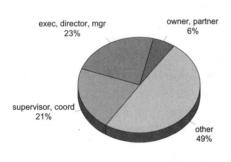

base: 10,829 practitioners

48% of RDs and 51% of DTRs reported they directly or indirectly supervise employees. For those supervising, the median number supervised is 8 for RDs and 15 for DTRs.

Exhibit 2.13

Number Supervised

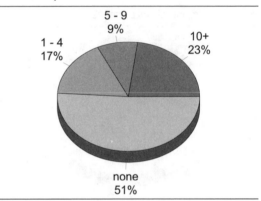

base: 10,829 practitioners

27% of RDs and 24% of DTRs reported managing a budget; for those doing so, the median budget size is $308,000 for RDs and $214,000 for DTRs, with 10% of RDs and 6% of DTRs managing budgets of $500,000 or more.

Exhibit 2.14

Budget Responsibility

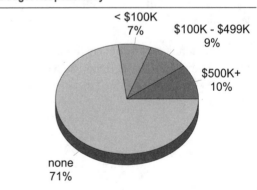

base: 10,829 practitioners

The typical practitioner has been in his or her primary dietetics position for 5 years, with 31% in the job for less than 3 years, and 33% in the job for 10 years or more.

Exhibit 2.15

Years in Position

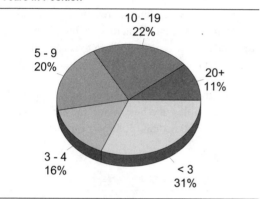

base: 10,829 practitioners

RD Compensation

64% of RDs reported their pay was based on 40 hours per week or more, with an additional 15% indicating a pay base of 30 to 39 hours per week. 88% of RDs indicated their position was year-round (52 weeks), with an additional 6% indicating pay based on 48 to 51 weeks per year.

In sum, 68% of practicing RDs reported working in their primary dietetics-related position full time (defined for the purposes of this survey as at least 35 hours per week for at least 48 weeks per year).

Exhibit 2.16

RD Pay Base

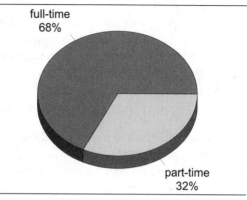

base: 8,621 answering RDs

(Analyses of hours worked and compensation received are based on the subset of respondents providing complete information for all relevant questions.)

Because the prevalence of part-time employment can make salary comparisons difficult, compensation is reported in two ways: in terms of *hourly wage,* and in terms of *total cash compensation* (which includes not only salary but also earnings from overtime pay, on-call pay, commissions, bonuses, incentive pay, profit sharing or distributions, and cash retirement benefits received — frequently important compensation components for consultants, executives, and those in sales positions). Hourly wage is assessed for all respondents; total cash compensation is examined only for those working full time for at least 1 year in the position.

Among all RDs in all positions, the median hourly wage as of April 1, 2002, was $22.00 per hour. If annualized (× 40 hours/week × 52 weeks/year), this equates to a full-time salary of $45,760 per year. Median total cash compensation for RDs employed in the position full time for at least 1 year was $45,800.

These results are higher than the most current Bureau of Labor Statistics (BLS) median wage estimate for Dietitians and Nutritionists of $18.48 per hour.[1] Two factors help account for the discrepancy: this survey data is current as of April 1, 2002, and is thus nearly two years more current than the BLS estimate; and BLS does not restrict its estimate to registered dietitians (virtually all survey respondents are registered).

Survey estimates are also higher than those found in the most recently published analysis of the ADA member database,[2] which reported an estimated median gross income for RDs of $40,450. Again, several factors help account for the variance: those data were collected for 1999; they were reported for full-time practitioners, but full time was defined more generously (31 hours per week or more); and a less precise compensation measure was employed.

The wide range of RD compensation is of interest:

Exhibit 2.17

RD Compensation

	Hourly Wage	Total Cash
10th percentile (10% earn less)	$16.20	$34,000
25th percentile (25% earn less)	$18.75	$38,900
50th percentile (50% earn less)	$22.00	$45,800
75th percentile (75% earn less)	$26.79	$56,000
90th percentile (90% earn less)	$33.65	$72,000

base: 8,621 answering RDs (hourly wage); 5,319 answering RDs (total cash compensation)

Helping to account for that range, a number of factors show strong associations with compensation levels for RDs. The following series of exhibits demonstrates the relationship between hourly wage and years in the field, years in the position, education, credentials, practice area, employer status, responsibility level, number supervised, budget responsibility, and location. Note that all factors are based on respondent self-reports and are thus subject to some variation in how terms were understood.

Bars on the charts are delimited by the 25th and 75th percentiles; the horizontal line across each bar marks the median (50th percentile).

Exhibit 2.18

RD Hourly Wage by Years in Field

	#	percentiles		
		25th	50th	75th
All RDs	8,621	$18.75	$22.00	$26.79
20+ years	3,110	$20.93	$24.89	$30.00
10 - 19 years	2,435	$19.74	$22.88	$27.43
5 - 9 years	1,501	$18.04	$20.50	$24.04
< 5 years	1,560	$16.01	$17.79	$20.19

NOTE: Years in field excludes time taken off to return to school, raise a family, or work in other areas.

As might be expected, years of dietetics experience is strongly associated with compensation; among practitioners with 20 or more years of experience, more than three-

[1] U.S. Department of Labor, Bureau of Labor Statistics. 2000 National Occupational Employment and Wage Estimates 29-1031 Dietitians and Nutritionists. http://www.bls.gov/oes/2000/oes291031.htm. Accessed 11/05/02.
[2] Bryk JA, Soto TK. Report on the 1999 membership database of the American Dietetic Association. *J Am Diet Assoc.* 2001;101:947-953.

fourths earn more than all but the top one-fourth of those with less than 5 years' experience.

Exhibit 2.19

RD Hourly Wage by Years in Position

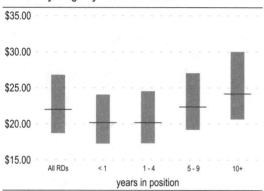

	percentiles		
	#	25th	50th	75th
All RDs	8,621	$18.75	$22.00	$26.79
10+ years	2,751	$20.67	$24.18	$30.00
5 - 9 years	1,720	$19.23	$22.36	$27.03
1 - 4 years	3,850	$17.37	$20.19	$24.52
< 1 year	279	$17.31	$20.19	$24.04

Entry-level wages (i.e., wages for individuals in the position less than 1 year) are not substantially different from those earned by practitioners with 1 to 4 years in the position. It is only with practitioners having a tenure of 5 years or more that material wage gains are observed.

Exhibit 2.20

RD Hourly Wage by Education Level

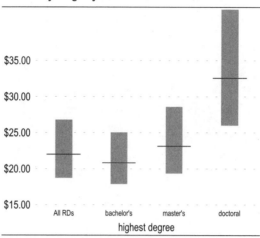

	percentiles		
	#	25th	50th	75th
All RDs	8,621	$18.75	$22.00	$26.79
doctoral degree	272	$26.04	$32.57	$42.06
master's degree	3,823	$19.39	$23.13	$28.57
bachelor's degree	4,497	$17.92	$20.83	$25.00

Education beyond the bachelor's degree is clearly associated with wage gains, though the effect is not uniform. Overall, the difference between the median wage of RDs with a bachelor's degree and that of RDs with a master's degree is $2.30; positions for which the differential associated with a master's degree exceeds that value include Clinical Dietitian, Long Term Care; Research Dietitian; School/Child Care Nutritionist; Executive-level Professional; Director of Food and Nutrition Services; Assistant Foodservice Director; and Director of Nutrition. Positions with below-average differentials for master's degrees are concentrated in the inpatient, outpatient, community, and business practice areas.

Exhibit 2.21

RD Hourly Wage by Credentials Held

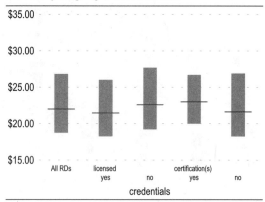

		percentiles		
	#	**25th**	**50th**	**75th**
All RDs	8,621	$18.75	$22.00	$26.79
state license	4,479	$18.27	$21.47	$26.00
no state license	4,142	$19.23	$22.60	$27.65
specialty certification(s)	1,420	$20.00	$23.00	$26.67
no certifications	7,201	$18.27	$21.63	$26.87

NOTE: Examples of specialty certifications provided to respondents included CNSD, CDE, FADA, CSR, CSP, CHE, CDM, CFPP, CFE, CFM.

Holding a state license is associated with somewhat lower compensation; however, this result could be due to the nature of positions requiring licensure and/or the general economic situation in states where licensure is in force.

Holding one or more specialty certifications is associated with an increased median wage, although the differential vanishes at the 75th percentile. The survey did not ask *which* specialty certifications were held, so the effect of any particular certification is unknown.

Exhibit 2.22

RD Hourly Wage by ADA Membership

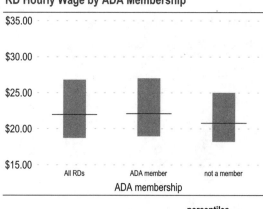

		percentiles		
	#	**25th**	**50th**	**75th**
All RDs	8,621	$18.75	$22.00	$26.79
ADA member	7,329	$18.99	$22.12	$27.00
not a member	1,292	$18.23	$20.81	$25.00

Results also show a small positive association between ADA membership and RD compensation.

Exhibit 2.23

RD Hourly Wage by Practice Area

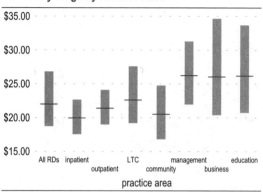

		percentiles		
	#	25th	50th	75th
All RDs	8,621	$18.75	$22.00	$26.79
acute care/inpatient	2,420	$17.55	$19.95	$22.62
ambulatory care	1,180	$18.99	$21.39	$24.07
long term care	1,020	$19.23	$22.61	$27.55
community	981	$16.83	$20.51	$24.73
food and nutrition management	1,198	$22.00	$26.22	$31.26
consultation and business	924	$20.43	$26.04	$34.62
education and research	539	$20.77	$26.17	$33.65

Wages tend to be highest in the practice areas of food and nutrition management, consultation and business, and education and research. Wages tend to be lower in the areas of acute care/inpatient, ambulatory care (outpatient), and community.

Exhibit 2.24

RD Hourly Wage by Employer Status

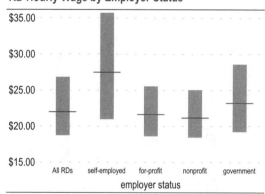

		percentiles		
	#	25th	50th	75th
All RDs	8,621	$18.75	$22.00	$26.79
self-employed	796	$21.00	$27.47	$35.69
for-profit	2,591	$18.63	$21.63	$25.50
nonprofit (other than government)	3,389	$18.46	$21.15	$25.00
government	1,704	$19.23	$23.20	$28.55

RDs self-employed in private practice or as consultants do markedly better than RDs in others' employ, on average. For those employed by others, median wages are highest for those working for the government, and lowest for those in nonprofit organizations.

Specific work settings for which median wages were highest included consultation or contract services to organizations, government agencies, school food service, contract food management companies, food manufacturers/distributors/retailers, and college or university faculty. Median wages were lowest in hospitals, clinics or ambulatory care centers, and community or public health programs.

Exhibit 2.25

RD Hourly Wage by Responsibility Level

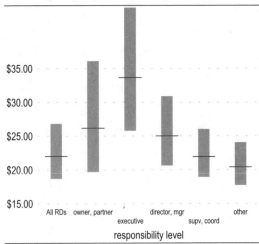

responsibility level

		percentiles		
	#	25th	50th	75th
All RDs	8,621	$18.75	$22.00	$26.79
owner or partner	440	$19.72	$26.15	$36.06
executive	143	$25.81	$33.65	$43.96
director or manager	1,955	$20.68	$25.00	$30.86
supervisor or coordinator	1,800	$18.99	$21.96	$26.00
other	4,173	$17.79	$20.43	$24.04

The relatively small cadre of executives reported exceptionally high hourly wages compared to all RDs, a disparity that increases more at the high end of the range when sources of compensation other than hourly wage (e.g., bonuses, incentive pay) are taken into account.

There is nearly a $5.00 per hour gap in median wage between those characterizing themselves as directors or managers, and those without supervisory or managerial responsibility.

Exhibit 2.26

RD Hourly Wage by Number Supervised

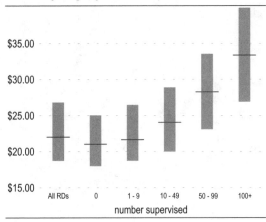

number supervised

		percentiles		
	#	25th	50th	75th
All RDs	8,621	$18.75	$22.00	$26.79
100+	203	$26.92	$33.33	$39.90
50 - 99	290	$23.08	$28.25	$33.51
10 - 49	1,399	$20.00	$24.04	$28.85
1 - 9	2,327	$18.75	$21.63	$26.44
0	4,377	$18.00	$21.01	$25.00

NOTE: includes employees supervised directly or indirectly

Supervisory responsibility is strongly associated with wage gains; those reporting direct and/or indirect supervision of 100 or more employees have a median wage more than 50% greater than the typical RD. These results closely mirror the results based on responsibility level, probably because wage levels tend to correspond to the position's rank in an organization's hierarchy.

Exhibit 2.27

RD Hourly Wage by Budget Responsibility

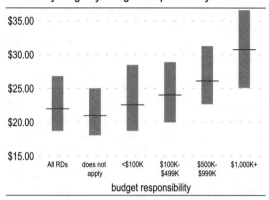

			percentiles	
	#	25th	50th	75th
All RDs	8,621	$18.75	$22.00	$26.79
$1,000K+	653	$25.13	$30.77	$36.56
$500K - $999K	299	$22.72	$26.11	$31.25
$100K - $499K	843	$20.00	$24.04	$28.85
< $100K	657	$18.75	$22.60	$28.44
does not apply	6,090	$18.10	$21.00	$25.00

Budget responsibility also correlates with wages, with gains increasing as budget size increases. Only about one-fourth of RDs manage budgets, however.

Exhibit 2.28

RD Hourly Wage by Location

(selected Census Divisions)

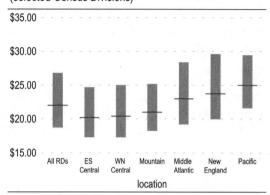

			percentiles	
	#	25th	50th	75th
All RDs	8,621	$18.75	$22.00	$26.79
East South Central	492	$17.32	$20.19	$24.67
West North Central	839	$17.31	$20.40	$25.00
Mountain	500	$18.27	$20.99	$25.18
Middle Atlantic	1,187	$19.23	$23.00	$28.37
New England	578	$20.00	$23.75	$29.58
Pacific	1,186	$21.63	$25.00	$29.43

RD compensation does vary by employment location. In terms of the nine standard Census Divisions, the East South Central states (Kentucky, Tennessee, Mississippi, Alabama), the West North Central states (North Dakota, South Dakota, Nebraska, Kansas, Minnesota, Iowa, Missouri), and the Mountain states (Idaho, Nevada, Utah, Arizona, Montana, Wyoming, Colorado, New Mexico) post below-average median wages, whereas the Middle Atlantic/New England states (Pennsylvania, New Jersey, New York, Connecticut, Rhode Island, Massachusetts, Vermont, New Hampshire, Maine) and Pacific states (Alaska, Hawaii, Washington, Oregon, California) post above-average median wages.

Further details of RD compensation by state and by major metropolitan area may be found in the *RD Compensation* section.

DTR Compensation

68% of DTRs reported their position's pay was based on 40 hours per week or more, with an additional 17% indicating a pay base of 30 to 39 hours per week. 96% indicated their position was essentially year-round (48 weeks per year or more).

In sum, 75% of DTRs work full time as defined in this report (35 hours or more per week for 48 weeks per year or more).

Exhibit 2.29
DTR Pay Base

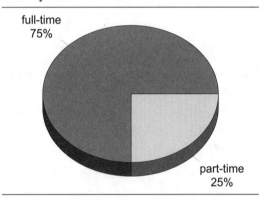

full-time 75%

part-time 25%

base: 1,397 answering DTRs

(Analyses of hours worked and compensation received are based on the subset of respondents providing complete information for all relevant questions.)

Among all DTRs in all positions, the median hourly wage as of April 1, 2002, was $14.74 per hour; if annualized, this equates to a salary of $30,660 per year. Median total cash compensation for DTRs employed in the position full time for at least 1 year was $31,000.

As with RDs, these current survey estimates are higher than those published by the Bureau of Labor Statistics (2000 median wage = $10.26)[3]

and in ADA's database analysis (1999 median gross income = $27,430) .[4] The factors previously discussed help to explain the discrepancies here, as well.

DTR compensation also spans a considerable range:

Exhibit 2.30
DTR Compensation

	Hourly Wage	Total Cash
10th percentile (10% earn less)	$11.31	$23,900
25th percentile (25% earn less)	$12.82	$27,000
50th percentile (50% earn less)	$14.74	$31,000
75th percentile (75% earn less)	$16.97	$36,300
90th percentile (90% earn less)	$20.19	$43,100

base: 1,397 answering DTRs (hourly wage); 938 answering DTRs (total cash compensation)

Helping to account for that range, a number of factors show strong associations with compensation levels for DTRs. The following series of exhibits demonstrates the relationship between hourly wage and years in the field, years in the position, education, credentials, practice area, employer status, responsibility level, number supervised, budget responsibility, and location. Note that all factors are based on respondent self-reports and are thus subject to some variation in how terms were understood.

[3] U.S. Department of Labor, Bureau of Labor Statistics. 2000 National Occupational Employment and Wage Estimates 29-2051 Dietetic Technicians.

http://www.bls.gov/oes/2000/oes292051.htm. Accessed 11/05/02.

[4] Bryk JA, Soto TK. Report on the 1999 membership database of the American Dietetic Association. *J Am Diet Assoc.* 2001;101:947-953.

Exhibit 2.31

DTR Hourly Wage by Years in Field

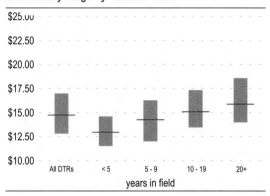

years in field

			percentiles	
	#	25th	50th	75th
All DTRs	1,397	$12.82	$14.74	$16.97
20+ years	336	$14.01	$15.87	$18.56
10 - 19 years	483	$13.46	$15.09	$17.31
5 - 9 years	353	$12.02	$14.26	$16.25
< 5 years	222	$11.54	$12.93	$14.58

DTR median wages show a steady increase with increasing experience, although the differential between those with fewer than 5 years of experience and those with 20 years or more is less than $3.00 per hour.

Exhibit 2.32

DTR Hourly Wage by Years in Position

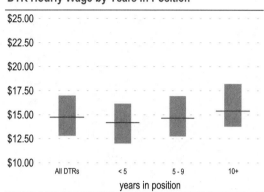

years in position

			percentiles	
	#	25th	50th	75th
All DTRs	1,397	$12.82	$14.74	$16.97
10+ years	479	$13.78	$15.39	$18.18
5 - 9 years	359	$12.75	$14.64	$16.92
< 5 years	558	$12.02	$14.18	$16.13

Similarly, the number of years in the specific position is clearly associated with compensation, although the effect is not great.

Exhibit 2.33

DTR Hourly Wage by Education Level

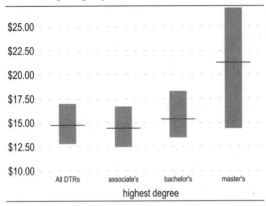

		percentiles		
	#	25th	50th	75th
All DTRs	1,397	$12.82	$14.74	$16.97
master's degree	35	$14.42	$21.25	$26.92
bachelor's degree	312	$13.46	$15.38	$18.27
associate's degree	1,048	$12.50	$14.42	$16.67

Those DTRs going beyond the required associate's degree to earn a bachelor's degree receive nearly an extra dollar per hour in median wage.

Exhibit 2.34

DTR Hourly Wage by Credentials Held

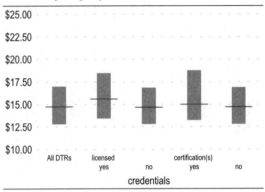

		percentiles		
	#	25th	50th	75th
All DTRs	1,397	$12.82	$14.74	$16.97
state license	83	$13.46	$15.60	$18.46
no state license	1,314	$12.82	$14.68	$16.83
specialty certification(s)	79	$13.28	$15.00	$18.75
no certifications	1,318	$12.82	$14.71	$16.87

NOTE: Examples of specialty certifications provided to respondents included CNSD, CDE, FADA, CSR, CSP, CHE, CDM, CFPP, CFE, CFM.

In reverse of the situation with RDs, the median wage of the small number of DTRs with a state license is almost a dollar an hour more than the median wage of those without. (Note that few states require DTRs to be licensed.) For DTRs, however, specialty certifications associate with little difference in median wage.

Exhibit 2.35

DTR Hourly Wage by ADA Membership

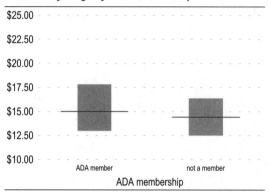

		percentiles		
	#	25th	50th	75th
All DTRs	1,397	$12.82	$14.74	$16.97
ADA member	769	$12.98	$15.00	$17.79
not a member	628	$12.51	$14.42	$16.35

As with RDs, ADA membership is associated with slightly higher compensation levels for DTRs.

Exhibit 2.36

DTR Hourly Wage by Practice Area

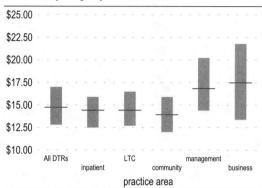

		percentiles		
	#	25th	50th	75th
All DTRs	1,397	$12.82	$14.74	$16.97
acute care/inpatient	561	$12.50	$14.42	$15.87
long term care	285	$12.71	$14.42	$16.46
community	139	$12.02	$13.94	$15.87
food and nutrition management	291	$14.42	$16.83	$20.19
consultation and business	30	$13.41	$17.47	$21.77

The median wage of DTRs holding positions in the practice areas of food and nutrition management and consultation and business is over $2.00 more per hour than the median wage of those in the inpatient, long term care, or community areas.

Exhibit 2.37

DTR Hourly Wage by Employer Status

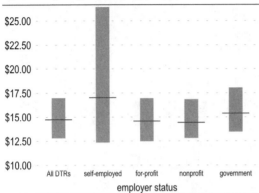

		percentiles		
	#	**25th**	**50th**	**75th**
All DTRs	1,397	$12.82	$14.74	$16.97
self-employed	26	$12.37	$17.03	$26.41
for-profit	446	$12.50	$14.57	$16.94
nonprofit	669	$12.82	$14.42	$16.83
government	223	$13.46	$15.38	$18.03

Self-employment is associated with a much greater range of DTR compensation than employment, although very few DTRs are self-employed. DTRs working for the government post slightly higher wages than those employed by for-profit or nonprofit organizations.

In terms of specific work settings, DTRs in school food service earn a median of $18.22 per hour, and those employed by a government agency earn a median of $17.31 per hour, whereas those working in hospitals or community/public health programs reported median wages of $14.42 and $13.90, respectively.

Exhibit 2.38

DTR Hourly Wage by Responsibility Level

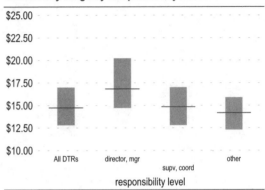

		percentiles		
	#	**25th**	**50th**	**75th**
All DTRs	1,397	$12.82	$14.74	$16.97
director or manager	295	$14.74	$16.83	$20.19
supervisor or coordinator	339	$12.82	$14.85	$16.99
other	733	$12.30	$14.18	$15.87

Responsibility level shows a clear association with DTR compensation, with those characterizing themselves as directors or managers earning a median wage $2.65 per hour higher than those without supervisory or management responsibility.

Exhibit 2.39

DTR Hourly Wage by Number Supervised

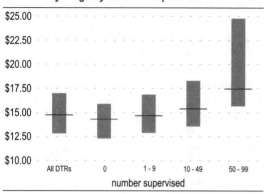

			percentiles	
	#	25th	50th	75th
All DTRs	1,397	$12.82	$14.74	$16.97
50 - 99	36	$15.69	$17.45	$24.76
10 - 49	422	$13.57	$15.38	$18.27
1 - 9	243	$12.88	$14.66	$16.83
0	668	$12.30	$14.28	$15.87

NOTE: Includes number of employees supervised directly or indirectly. Results for supervision of 100 or more employees not shown due to insufficient response.

Reflecting essentially the same phenomenon, DTR compensation is strongly associated with supervisory responsibility, especially as the number supervised grows larger.

Exhibit 2.40

DTR Hourly Wage by Budget Responsibility

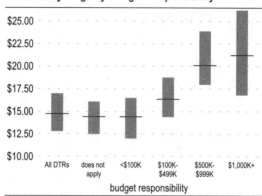

			percentiles	
	#	25th	50th	75th
All DTRs	1,397	$12.82	$14.74	$16.97
$1,000K+	47	$16.83	$21.20	$26.20
$500K - $999K	42	$17.99	$20.09	$23.87
$100K - $499K	159	$14.42	$16.35	$18.75
< $100K	90	$12.02	$14.42	$16.48
does not apply	995	$12.50	$14.42	$16.07

Budget responsibility is also clearly associated with DTR compensation, although the differentials between no budget responsibility and responsibility for small budgets (under $100,000) are minimal.

Exhibit 2.41

DTR Hourly Wage by Location

(selected Census Divisions)

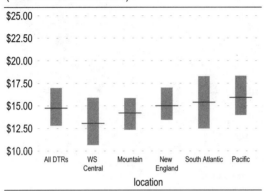

	#	percentiles		
		25th	50th	75th
All DTRs	1,397	$12.82	$14.74	$16.97
West South Central	52	$10.68	$13.05	$15.89
Mountain	34	$12.36	$14.20	$15.85
New England	119	$13.46	$15.00	$17.00
South Atlantic	183	$12.50	$15.38	$18.27
Pacific	136	$13.99	$15.93	$18.31

As with RD compensation, median DTR wages do vary by employment location. DTRs in the West South Central states (Oklahoma, Texas, Arkansas, Louisiana) and the Mountain states (Idaho, Nevada, Utah, Arizona, Montana, Wyoming, Colorado, New Mexico) earn median wages significantly below the median for all DTRs, while those in the New England (Maine, Vermont, New Hampshire, Massachusetts, Connecticut, Rhode Island), South Atlantic (West Virginia, Maryland, Delaware, District of Columbia, Virginia, North Carolina, South Carolina, Georgia, Florida) and Pacific (Alaska, Hawaii, Washington, Oregon, California) states earn more.

Compensation By Position

As noted previously, survey respondents were asked to match their job to one of 58 core position descriptions developed by the ADA, regardless of whether the position title was similar to their own. 95% of respondents selected one of the standard positions, indicating that survey results represent the vast majority of dietetics employment situations.

The following exhibits report hourly wages at the 25th, 50th and 75th percentiles for all positions returning sufficient numbers of responses. Further results showing how compensation is related to a variety of factors, and additionally reporting total cash compensation, may be found in the *Compensation by Position* section.

Exhibit 2.42

Hourly Wage: Positions in the Clinical Nutrition — Acute Care/Inpatient Practice Area

	#	percentiles		
		25th	50th	75th
Dietetic Technician, Clinical	553	$12.45	$14.42	$15.87
Clinical Dietitian	1,462	$17.03	$19.23	$22.00
Clinical Dietitian, Specialist — Cardiac	63	$17.31	$19.13	$20.19
Clinical Dietitian, Specialist — Diabetes	136	$18.30	$20.67	$24.04
Clinical Dietitian, Specialist — Oncology	70	$16.96	$19.60	$22.60
Clinical Dietitian, Specialist — Renal	216	$19.23	$21.15	$24.00
Clinical Dietitian, Specialist — Other	141	$18.27	$20.19	$23.08
Pediatric/Neonatal Dietitian	165	$17.50	$19.71	$22.20
Nutrition Support Dietitian	202	$19.66	$21.79	$24.72

Exhibit 2.43

Hourly Wage: Positions in the Clinical Nutrition — Ambulatory Care Practice Area

	#	percentiles		
		25th	50th	75th
Outpatient Dietitian, General	332	$18.20	$20.99	$24.06
Outpatient Dietitian, Specialist — Cardiac Rehabilitation	39	$18.13	$19.39	$23.21
Outpatient Dietitian, Specialist — Diabetes	345	$19.23	$21.15	$24.04
Outpatient Dietitian, Specialist — Pediatrics	59	$18.99	$22.05	$24.57
Outpatient Dietitian, Specialist — Renal	245	$19.86	$22.00	$24.39
Outpatient Dietitian, Specialist — Weight Management	55	$17.31	$19.23	$21.63
Outpatient Dietitian, Specialist — Other	51	$18.03	$22.00	$25.00
Home Care Dietitian	68	$20.00	$24.43	$27.50

Exhibit 2.44

Hourly Wage: Positions in the Clinical Nutrition — Long Term Care Practice Area

	#	percentiles		
		25th	50th	75th
Clinical Dietitian, Long Term Care	1,084	$18.99	$21.99	$26.92
Dietetic Technician, Long Term Care	232	$12.50	$14.25	$15.91

Exhibit 2.45

Hourly Wage: Positions in the Community Practice Area

	#	25th	50th	75th
			percentiles	
WIC Nutritionist	585	$15.14	$17.79	$21.59
Public Health Nutritionist	317	$18.44	$22.60	$27.32
Cooperative Extension Educator/Specialist	87	$15.00	$19.23	$24.04
School/Child Care Nutritionist	71	$18.27	$26.44	$31.89
Nutrition Coordinator for Head Start Program	36	$13.98	$18.09	$22.11
Nutritionist for Food Bank or Assistance Program	26	$15.38	$17.00	$21.46

Exhibit 2.46

Hourly Wage: Positions in the Food and Nutrition Management Practice Area

	#	25th	50th	75th
			percentiles	
Executive-level Professional	193	$28.85	$34.86	$41.80
Director of Food and Nutrition Services	579	$20.19	$25.07	$30.55
Clinical Nutrition Manager	336	$21.67	$25.00	$28.08
Assistant Foodservice Director	131	$18.27	$21.63	$25.96
School Foodservice Director	116	$20.20	$24.83	$30.40
Dietetic Technician, Foodservice Management	155	$13.46	$15.38	$18.43

Exhibit 2.47

Hourly Wage: Positions in the Consultation and Business Practice Area

	#	25th	50th	75th
			percentiles	
Private Practice Dietitian — Patient/Client Nutrition Care	258	$16.90	$24.04	$34.34
Consultation — Community and/or Corporate Programs	153	$19.11	$25.00	$33.15
Consultant — Communications	74	$20.11	$25.73	$39.15
Sales Representative	192	$22.26	$25.96	$32.80
Public Relations and/or Marketing Professional	38	$23.56	$29.43	$36.54
Corporate Dietitian	66	$17.79	$22.48	$28.85
Research & Development Nutritionist	37	$21.88	$30.30	$37.93
Manager of Nutrition Communications	46	$20.49	$24.67	$33.95
Director of Nutrition	99	$24.04	$29.23	$39.42

Exhibit 2.48

Hourly Wage: Positions in the Education and Research Practice Area

		percentiles		
	#	25th	50th	75th
Instructor/Lecturer	128	$19.24	$22.91	$30.04
Assistant Professor	56	$25.04	$29.75	$32.82
Associate Professor	58	$27.66	$31.25	$36.70
Professor	43	$34.72	$40.48	$51.83
Administrator, Higher Education	27	$35.10	$43.85	$50.48
Dietetic Internship Director	52	$21.81	$24.51	$27.64
Research Dietitian	175	$17.79	$21.15	$26.44

Benefits

Although many are employed part-time, dietetics practitioners as a group enjoy considerable fringe benefits from their work. 81% receive paid vacation or personal time off, 75% paid holidays, and 74% paid sick days. 81% have some sort of medical coverage, compared to only 64% of a reference group of US professional/technical employees in private industry.[5] 73% have dental coverage and 54% have vision coverage, well above the reference group values of 42% and 24%, respectively. 68% of dietetics professionals receive a prescription drug benefit.

70% receive life insurance, and 61% some form of disability insurance. 63% reported participation in defined contribution retirement programs (such as 401[k] plans), compared to 53% of the reference group, whereas 45% participate in defined benefit (pension) retirement programs, compared to only 27% of the reference group.

59% receive funding for professional development (conferences, seminars, etc.), and 22% have their professional society dues paid. 42% receive assistance with college tuition. 41% have access to an employee assistance or wellness program. 35% work with comp time or flex time. 29% receive a fitness benefit such as a discounted health club membership or an on-site facility. 26% are eligible for extended and/or paid maternity leave, and 12% have on-site child care or a child care allowance.

Benefit levels are most influenced by employment status (self-employed versus not; full-time versus part-time). Those working in hospitals, schools, or government agencies tend to enjoy a richer array of benefits than those employed in other areas, particularly extended care.

---

[5] U.S. Department of Labor, Bureau of Labor Statistics. Employee Benefits in Private Industry, 2000. http://www.bls.gov/news.release/ebs2.nr0.htm. Accessed 11/05/02.

Exhibit 2.49

Benefits Offered As Part of Employment/Self-Employment

	%
NET: paid time off	83%
paid vacation, personal time off	81%
paid holidays	75%
paid sick days	74%
NET: medical	81%
medical insurance, group plan, or savings account	81%
dental insurance or group plan	73%
prescription drug benefit	68%
vision insurance or group plan	54%
NET: insurance	74%
life insurance	70%
disability insurance (long- and/or short-term)	61%
NET: retirement, investments	76%
defined contribution retirement plan (e.g., 401[k], SEP)	63%
defined benefit retirement plan (pension)	45%
stock options, ESOP	9%
profit sharing	8%
NET: professional development	61%
funding for professional development (conferences, seminars, etc.)	59%
professional society dues	22%
NET: quality of work life	72%
college tuition assistance	42%
employee assistance or wellness program	41%
comp time or flex time	35%
fitness benefit (e.g., discounted health club membership, on-site facilities)	29%
extended and/or paid parental leave	26%
on-site child care or allowance	12%
telecommuting	7%
other	3%
indicated one or more	89%
no benefits	10%
no answer	1%

base: 10,829 practitioners (multiple answers)

Conclusion

As the most comprehensive survey of compensation in the dietetics profession to date, the *ADA 2002 Dietetics Compensation & Benefits Survey* provides new perspectives on how specific dietetics jobs are compensated, and how a variety of factors relate to compensation levels. ADA plans to periodically update the survey and actively seeks suggestions for its improvement. With the help and participation of dietetics professionals, future surveys can become even more of an asset to the profession.

3. RD Compensation

Notes

Tables in this section report compensation for the 8,621 Registered Dietitians (RDs) who provided complete hour and compensation information. Results are broken out by a number of factors to demonstrate the relative effects of qualifications, experience, and employment situation in determining compensation levels.

Note that all factors are based on respondent self-reports and are thus subject to some variation in how terms were understood.

Two measures are reported: *hourly wage* and *total cash compensation*.

In accordance with Bureau of Labor Statistics practice, hourly wage may be converted to an annualized salary by multiplying the wage by 40 hours per week and 52 weeks per year.

Total cash compensation is reported only for practitioners employed or self-employed in the position full time for at least 1 year, and includes sources of compensation beyond salary/wages, such as bonuses, commissions, on-call pay, etc. For some workers, such as consultants, salespeople, and executives, a significant part of their compensation can come from sources other than salary. For such individuals, total cash compensation provides a more accurate picture of compensation than wages alone.

In addition to the number of individuals answering, 5 percentile values are reported for each measure: 10% of practitioners earn less than the 10th percentile, 25% earn less than the 25th percentile, and so on. All percentiles are suppressed if there are fewer than 25 valid responses; the 10th and 90th percentiles are suppressed if there are fewer than 50 valid responses.

Compensation by location is reported in terms of the nine standard Census Divisions:

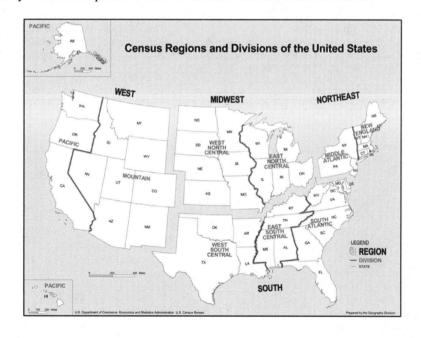

Census Regions and Divisions of the United States

Exhibit 3.1

RD Compensation by Years in Field

| | # answering | HOURLY WAGE | | | | | # answering | TOTAL CASH COMPENSATION (those employed full time, 1+ years) | | | | |
| | | percentiles | | | | | | percentiles | | | | |
		10th	25th	50th	75th	90th		10th	25th	50th	75th	90th
All RDs	8621	$16.20	$18.75	$22.00	$26.79	$33.65	5319	$34,000	$38,900	$45,800	$56,000	$72,000
Years In Field												
20+ years	3110	$18.27	$20.93	$24.89	$30.00	$37.95	1904	$40,000	$45,000	$52,700	$65,000	$82,300
10 - 19 years	2435	$17.31	$19.74	$22.88	$27.43	$33.65	1354	$36,600	$41,100	$48,000	$57,000	$72,000
5 - 9 years	1501	$16.22	$18.04	$20.50	$24.04	$28.85	923	$34,000	$37,700	$42,800	$51,000	$60,500
< 5 years	1560	$14.79	$16.01	$17.79	$20.19	$24.00	1129	$30,800	$33,400	$37,000	$41,600	$47,800

Note: Results not shown if fewer than 25 valid values; 10th and 90th percentiles not shown if fewer than 50 valid values.

Exhibit 3.2

RD Compensation by Years in Position

| | # answering | HOURLY WAGE | | | | | # answering | TOTAL CASH COMPENSATION (those employed full time, 1+ years) | | | | |
| | | percentiles | | | | | | percentiles | | | | |
		10th	25th	50th	75th	90th		10th	25th	50th	75th	90th
All RDs	8621	$16.20	$18.75	$22.00	$26.79	$33.65	5319	$34,000	$38,900	$45,800	$56,000	$72,000
Years In Position												
10+ years	2751	$18.34	$20.67	$24.18	$30.00	$38.46	1753	$39,300	$44,000	$51,000	$62,900	$82,000
5 - 9 years	1720	$16.83	$19.23	$22.36	$27.03	$33.65	1017	$35,000	$40,000	$46,000	$56,100	$70,000
1 - 4 years	3850	$15.38	$17.37	$20.19	$24.52	$29.91	2549	$32,100	$36,000	$41,600	$51,000	$62,500
< 1 year	279	$15.27	$17.31	$20.19	$24.04	$29.45						

Note: Results not shown if fewer than 25 valid values; 10th and 90th percentiles not shown if fewer than 50 valid values.

Exhibit 3.3

RD Compensation by Education

	# answering	HOURLY WAGE percentiles					# answering	TOTAL CASH COMPENSATION (those employed full time, 1+ years) percentiles				
		10th	25th	50th	75th	90th		10th	25th	50th	75th	90th
All RDs	8621	$16.20	$18.75	$22.00	$26.79	$33.65	5319	$34,000	$38,900	$45,800	$56,000	$72,000
Education (Highest Degree)												
doctoral degree	272	$20.19	$26.04	$32.57	$42.06	$51.89	149	$44,000	$55,000	$70,100	$95,000	$115,000
master's degree	3823	$16.83	$19.39	$23.13	$28.57	$35.10	2350	$36,000	$40,700	$49,000	$60,000	$76,000
bachelor's degree	4497	$15.57	$17.92	$20.83	$25.00	$30.00	2801	$32,900	$37,000	$43,000	$52,000	$62,500
associate's degree	7						7					

Note: Results not shown if fewer than 25 valid values; 10th and 90th percentiles not shown if fewer than 50 valid values.

Exhibit 3.4

RD Compensation by Education and Years in Field

	# answering	HOURLY WAGE percentiles					# answering	TOTAL CASH COMPENSATION (those employed full time, 1+ years) percentiles				
		10th	25th	50th	75th	90th		10th	25th	50th	75th	90th
All RDs	8621	$16.20	$18.75	$22.00	$26.79	$33.65	5319	$34,000	$38,900	$45,800	$56,000	$72,000
doctoral degree	272	$20.19	$26.04	$32.57	$42.06	$51.89	149	$44,000	$55,000	$70,100	$95,000	$115,000
20+ years	155	$22.69	$28.85	$36.81	$47.12	$55.05	86	$54,700	$64,800	$82,000	$107,100	$132,300
10 - 19 years	78	$20.83	$24.28	$29.36	$37.56	$45.06	43		$51,800	$62,900	$78,300	
5 - 9 years	23						7					
< 5 years	15						13					
master's degree	3823	$16.83	$19.39	$23.13	$28.57	$35.10	2350	$36,000	$40,700	$49,000	$60,000	$76,000
20+ years	1582	$18.75	$21.32	$25.47	$30.86	$37.50	1002	$40,300	$46,200	$54,500	$67,800	$82,000
10 - 19 years	1164	$17.79	$20.00	$23.59	$28.65	$35.00	665	$38,000	$41,800	$49,200	$60,000	$75,000
5 - 9 years	555	$16.83	$18.99	$21.63	$25.48	$31.42	324	$35,000	$39,500	$45,000	$54,000	$63,400
< 5 years	514	$15.33	$16.81	$18.29	$21.32	$24.76	354	$32,000	$34,800	$38,000	$42,900	$49,700
bachelor's degree	4497	$15.57	$17.92	$20.83	$25.00	$30.00	2801	$32,900	$37,000	$43,000	$52,000	$62,500
20+ years	1365	$17.89	$20.20	$23.47	$28.17	$34.62	813	$38,500	$43,100	$50,000	$59,200	$74,900
10 - 19 years	1184	$17.03	$19.23	$21.88	$25.72	$31.51	638	$36,000	$40,300	$45,700	$53,000	$65,000
5 - 9 years	919	$15.87	$17.55	$20.00	$23.22	$26.92	591	$33,300	$37,000	$41,600	$49,800	$58,000
< 5 years	1023	$14.42	$15.87	$17.50	$19.88	$23.08	755	$30,100	$33,000	$36,500	$41,000	$47,000

Note: Results not shown if fewer than 25 valid values; 10th and 90th percentiles not shown if fewer than 50 valid values.

Exhibit 3.5

RD Compensation by Credentials Held

| | # answering | HOURLY WAGE | | | | | # answering | TOTAL CASH COMPENSATION (those employed full time, 1+ years) | | | | |
		10th	25th	50th	75th	90th		10th	25th	50th	75th	90th
All RDs	8621	$16.20	$18.75	$22.00	$26.79	$33.65	5319	$34,000	$38,900	$45,800	$56,000	$72,000
Credentials Held												
state license	4479	$15.87	$18.27	$21.47	$26.00	$32.90	2795	$33,500	$38,000	$45,000	$54,400	$68,000
no state license	4142	$16.39	$19.23	$22.60	$27.65	$34.71	2524	$34,500	$40,000	$47,000	$58,000	$75,000
specialty certification(s)	1420	$18.03	$20.00	$23.00	$26.67	$32.68	879	$37,100	$41,600	$48,100	$56,200	$69,000
no specialty certification	7201	$15.87	$18.27	$21.63	$26.87	$33.97	4440	$33,300	$38,000	$45,000	$56,000	$72,200

Note: Results not shown if fewer than 25 valid values; 10th and 90th percentiles not shown if fewer than 50 valid values.

Exhibit 3.6

RD Compensation by ADA Membership

| | # answering | HOURLY WAGE | | | | | # answering | TOTAL CASH COMPENSATION (those employed full time, 1+ years) | | | | |
		10th	25th	50th	75th	90th		10th	25th	50th	75th	90th
All RDs	8621	$16.20	$18.75	$22.00	$26.79	$33.65	5319	$34,000	$38,900	$45,800	$56,000	$72,000
ADA Membership												
ADA member	7329	$16.35	$18.99	$22.12	$27.00	$34.07	4532	$34,200	$39,100	$46,300	$57,000	$72,300
not a member	1292	$15.60	$18.23	$20.81	$25.00	$31.40	787	$32,700	$37,000	$43,000	$52,000	$68,000

Note: Results not shown if fewer than 25 valid values; 10th and 90th percentiles not shown if fewer than 50 valid values.

Exhibit 3.7

RD Compensation by Practice Area

| | HOURLY WAGE | | | | | | TOTAL CASH COMPENSATION (those employed full time, 1+ years) | | | | | |
| | # answering | 10th | 25th | 50th | 75th | 90th | # answering | 10th | 25th | 50th | 75th | 90th |
		------- percentiles -------						------- percentiles -------				
All RDs	8621	$16.20	$18.75	$22.00	$26.79	$33.65	5319	$34,000	$38,900	$45,800	$56,000	$72,000
Practice Area												
clinical nutrition — acute care/inpatient	2420	$15.75	$17.55	$19.95	$22.62	$25.79	1568	$32,500	$36,000	$40,800	$46,900	$53,000
clinical nutrition — ambulatory care	1180	$16.78	$18.99	$21.39	$24.07	$27.40	580	$34,700	$38,300	$44,000	$50,000	$57,000
clinical nutrition — long term care	1020	$16.67	$19.23	$22.61	$27.55	$35.00	520	$34,000	$38,100	$43,300	$50,500	$60,500
community	981	$14.90	$16.83	$20.51	$24.73	$29.81	661	$31,200	$35,500	$43,200	$51,500	$62,000
food and nutrition management	1198	$19.17	$22.00	$26.22	$31.26	$37.50	1013	$40,000	$47,000	$55,000	$67,300	$82,000
consultation and business	924	$15.87	$20.43	$26.04	$34.62	$43.63	506	$38,400	$46,800	$60,000	$78,600	$100,600
education and research	539	$17.09	$20.77	$26.17	$33.65	$44.63	236	$36,700	$43,600	$54,800	$70,100	$95,900

Note: Results not shown if fewer than 25 valid values; 10th and 90th percentiles not shown if fewer than 50 valid values.

Exhibit 3.8

RD Compensation by Practice Area and Years in Field

| | | HOURLY WAGE | | | | | | TOTAL CASH COMPENSATION (those employed full time, 1+ years) | | | | |
	# answering	10th	25th	50th	75th	90th	# answering	10th	25th	50th	75th	90th
All RDs	8621	$16.20	$18.75	$22.00	$26.79	$33.65	5319	$34,000	$38,900	$45,800	$56,000	$72,000
clinical nutrition — acute care/inpatient	2420	$15.75	$17.55	$19.95	$22.62	$25.79	1568	$32,500	$36,000	$40,800	$46,900	$53,000
20+ years	678	$18.27	$19.79	$22.00	$24.67	$28.04	413	$38,100	$41,700	$46,500	$51,400	$57,700
10 - 19 years	617	$17.31	$19.23	$20.71	$23.39	$26.18	348	$36,000	$39,700	$43,300	$48,600	$54,000
5 - 9 years	456	$15.75	$17.31	$19.23	$21.35	$24.04	286	$32,900	$36,000	$40,000	$44,500	$50,400
< 5 years	664	$14.81	$15.85	$17.31	$19.23	$21.70	518	$30,700	$33,000	$36,000	$39,600	$43,500
clinical nutrition — ambulatory care	1180	$16.78	$18.99	$21.39	$24.07	$27.40	580	$34,700	$38,300	$44,000	$50,000	$57,000
20+ years	404	$18.27	$20.51	$22.73	$25.31	$28.31	193	$38,000	$43,600	$47,500	$54,700	$59,700
10 - 19 years	344	$17.80	$19.84	$22.12	$25.00	$28.67	140	$36,800	$40,100	$46,000	$51,300	$56,000
5 - 9 years	222	$16.83	$18.28	$20.02	$22.23	$25.08	113	$35,000	$38,200	$40,600	$46,000	$51,200
< 5 years	207	$14.95	$16.48	$18.00	$21.15	$23.57	131	$31,200	$34,000	$37,000	$42,000	$49,900
clinical nutrition — long term care	1020	$16.67	$19.23	$22.61	$27.55	$35.00	520	$34,000	$38,100	$43,300	$50,500	$60,500
20+ years	346	$17.77	$20.95	$25.14	$32.01	$37.89	152	$39,400	$44,000	$50,000	$58,000	$72,000
10 - 19 years	281	$17.79	$19.84	$23.44	$29.43	$37.42	122	$35,500	$39,900	$43,600	$51,000	$62,400
5 - 9 years	200	$16.83	$19.23	$21.63	$25.00	$28.85	113	$35,000	$38,800	$43,700	$49,000	$56,200
< 5 years	190	$15.38	$16.65	$18.99	$21.27	$24.50	132	$32,000	$34,500	$38,500	$42,000	$45,700
community	981	$14.90	$16.83	$20.51	$24.73	$29.81	661	$31,200	$35,500	$43,200	$51,500	$62,000
20+ years	343	$16.49	$19.75	$23.25	$28.37	$33.27	235	$36,000	$43,000	$50,000	$59,000	$71,600
10 - 19 years	291	$15.38	$17.31	$20.78	$24.97	$29.81	192	$32,100	$36,700	$43,200	$51,000	$62,100
5 - 9 years	165	$14.90	$16.35	$18.65	$23.04	$27.46	106	$31,400	$33,800	$38,800	$45,400	$55,000
< 5 years	181	$13.46	$15.06	$16.83	$19.86	$22.94	127	$28,400	$31,000	$35,000	$41,600	$47,600
food and nutrition management	1198	$19.17	$22.00	$26.22	$31.26	$37.50	1013	$40,000	$47,000	$55,000	$67,300	$82,000
20+ years	615	$21.10	$24.60	$28.85	$34.23	$40.38	532	$45,300	$52,000	$60,000	$74,000	$89,000
10 - 19 years	335	$19.24	$22.16	$25.50	$30.77	$35.19	271	$41,000	$47,700	$54,000	$65,000	$77,500
5 - 9 years	162	$17.46	$19.98	$23.53	$26.68	$30.74	139	$36,700	$42,600	$50,000	$56,000	$65,000
< 5 years	86	$15.31	$16.83	$19.03	$21.17	$22.33	71	$32,000	$35,000	$39,000	$43,200	$47,400
consultation and business	924	$15.87	$20.43	$26.04	$34.62	$43.63	506	$38,400	$46,800	$60,000	$78,600	$100,600
20+ years	311	$15.43	$21.70	$28.85	$37.50	$48.03	157	$40,200	$54,900	$70,000	$90,000	$119,500
10 - 19 years	307	$16.87	$22.12	$27.64	$35.58	$43.66	161	$42,000	$49,800	$62,000	$81,000	$104,000
5 - 9 years	171	$17.40	$21.15	$24.52	$33.33	$40.31	95	$42,200	$51,300	$61,200	$75,000	$92,000
< 5 years	134	$15.38	$17.19	$20.44	$25.00	$36.13	93	$32,000	$36,000	$43,000	$52,800	$75,100
education and research	539	$17.09	$20.77	$26.17	$33.65	$44.63	236	$36,700	$43,600	$54,800	$70,100	$95,900
20+ years	259	$19.06	$24.04	$29.81	$38.46	$50.00	116	$44,000	$52,000	$64,500	$83,000	$109,300
10 - 19 years	151	$19.23	$21.63	$26.44	$31.25	$38.59	53	$42,200	$47,500	$55,600	$66,700	$89,000
5 - 9 years	74	$16.83	$19.00	$22.50	$28.05	$35.54	37		$37,800	$43,500	$53,500	
< 5 years	53	$14.94	$15.95	$18.63	$21.75	$27.34	29		$34,700	$38,800	$43,100	

Note: Results not shown if fewer than 25 valid values; 10th and 90th percentiles not shown if fewer than 50 valid values.

Exhibit 3.9

RD Compensation by Employment Setting

| | | HOURLY WAGE | | | | | | TOTAL CASH COMPENSATION (those employed full time, 1+ years) | | | | |
| | # answering | 10th | 25th | 50th | 75th | 90th | # answering | 10th | 25th | 50th | 75th | 90th |
		-------- percentiles --------						-------- percentiles --------				
All RDs	8621	$16.20	$18.75	$22.00	$26.79	$33.65	5319	$34,000	$38,900	$45,800	$56,000	$72,000
Employment Setting private practice or												
consultation to individuals	286	$11.66	$17.88	$23.42	$30.35	$42.35	60	$20,200	$35,000	$44,800	$60,000	$99,000
consultation or contract services to organizations	577	$16.80	$20.64	$25.84	$33.33	$41.67	192	$36,000	$42,000	$50,000	$64,800	$80,000
hospital	2919	$16.02	$18.11	$20.62	$24.28	$28.94	2033	$33,300	$37,700	$43,200	$52,000	$63,000
clinic or ambulatory care center	852	$17.16	$19.23	$21.63	$24.39	$27.11	466	$35,600	$39,500	$45,000	$51,000	$56,800
extended care facility	889	$16.83	$19.23	$22.44	$26.92	$34.19	539	$35,000	$39,400	$45,000	$52,000	$63,000
managed care organization, physician, other provider	131	$16.05	$19.33	$22.12	$26.44	$28.90	73	$33,400	$39,500	$48,000	$58,200	$64,000
community or public health program	819	$14.50	$16.57	$20.00	$24.04	$28.27	541	$31,000	$35,000	$42,000	$50,000	$59,000
government agency	379	$16.79	$19.89	$24.23	$30.00	$37.62	317	$35,000	$41,300	$50,000	$62,200	$77,800
school food service	194	$17.56	$20.43	$26.18	$31.75	$37.22	109	$38,500	$44,700	$56,500	$69,000	$81,000
contract food management company	175	$17.79	$19.58	$25.48	$30.29	$38.65	152	$38,000	$41,800	$54,000	$68,500	$97,900
food manufacturer, distributor, retailer	159	$17.98	$21.50	$26.44	$34.62	$43.27	138	$40,000	$49,800	$64,000	$86,500	$105,300
college or university faculty	426	$17.72	$22.12	$27.50	$35.61	$45.75	169	$38,800	$46,700	$55,500	$74,500	$102,400

Note: Results not shown if fewer than 25 valid values; 10th and 90th percentiles not shown if fewer than 50 valid values.

Exhibit 3.10

RD Compensation by Employer Status

	# answering	HOURLY WAGE					# answering	TOTAL CASH COMPENSATION (those employed full time, 1+ years)				
		percentiles						percentiles				
		10th	25th	50th	75th	90th		10th	25th	50th	75th	90th
All RDs	8621	$16.20	$18.75	$22.00	$26.79	$33.65	5319	$34,000	$38,900	$45,800	$56,000	$72,000
Employer Status												
self-employed	796	$15.00	$21.00	$27.47	$35.69	$43.27	147	$31,900	$45,000	$55,000	$75,000	$93,000
for-profit	2591	$16.35	$18.63	$21.63	$25.50	$31.73	1728	$34,100	$38,600	$45,600	$57,200	$76,300
nonprofit												
(other than government)	3389	$16.18	$18.46	$21.15	$25.00	$30.82	2151	$33,700	$38,100	$44,300	$53,000	$65,000
government	1704	$16.34	$19.23	$23.20	$28.55	$34.62	1224	$34,500	$40,000	$49,000	$59,000	$73,300

Note: Results not shown if fewer than 25 valid values; 10th and 90th percentiles not shown if fewer than 50 valid values.

Exhibit 3.11

RD Compensation by Size of Organization

	# answering	HOURLY WAGE					# answering	TOTAL CASH COMPENSATION (those employed full time, 1+ years)				
		percentiles						percentiles				
		10th	25th	50th	75th	90th		10th	25th	50th	75th	90th
All RDs	8621	$16.20	$18.75	$22.00	$26.79	$33.65	5319	$34,000	$38,900	$45,800	$56,000	$72,000
Size of Organization (Number Employed)												
1,000 or more	3553	$16.67	$19.23	$22.13	$27.01	$33.74	2476	$34,800	$40,000	$47,300	$60,000	$77,400
100 - 999	2478	$16.49	$18.75	$21.63	$25.96	$31.03	1614	$34,500	$39,000	$45,000	$54,300	$65,400
10 - 99	1189	$15.38	$17.64	$20.67	$24.94	$29.86	742	$31,800	$36,100	$43,200	$52,000	$62,500
2 - 9	457	$14.90	$17.26	$20.00	$24.21	$31.90	257	$32,100	$36,000	$41,500	$49,300	$61,300
1 (self-employed)	686	$14.67	$20.98	$27.01	$35.52	$42.67	113	$33,100	$44,500	$52,000	$70,000	$91,200

Note: Results not shown if fewer than 25 valid values; 10th and 90th percentiles not shown if fewer than 50 valid values.

Exhibit 3.12

RD Compensation by Responsibility Level

	# answering	HOURLY WAGE percentiles					# answering	TOTAL CASH COMPENSATION (those employed full time, 1+ years) percentiles				
		10th	25th	50th	75th	90th		10th	25th	50th	75th	90th
All RDs	8621	$16.20	$18.75	$22.00	$26.79	$33.65	5319	$34,000	$38,900	$45,800	$56,000	$72,000
Responsibility Level												
owner or partner	440	$12.50	$19.72	$26.15	$36.06	$45.82	125	$30,400	$40,800	$58,000	$77,000	$100,000
executive	143	$20.29	$25.81	$33.65	$43.96	$54.35	121	$43,100	$56,000	$77,600	$104,000	$134,600
director or manager	1955	$18.12	$20.68	$25.00	$30.86	$37.50	1591	$38,000	$44,000	$53,000	$65,900	$81,000
supervisor or coordinator	1800	$16.59	$18.99	$21.96	$26.00	$31.25	1143	$34,500	$39,000	$45,000	$53,400	$62,500
other	4173	$15.59	$17.79	$20.43	$24.04	$28.94	2290	$32,400	$36,000	$41,800	$49,400	$58,000

Note: Results not shown if fewer than 25 valid values; 10th and 90th percentiles not shown if fewer than 50 valid values.

Exhibit 3.13

RD Compensation by Number Supervised

	# answering	HOURLY WAGE percentiles					# answering	TOTAL CASH COMPENSATION (those employed full time, 1+ years) percentiles				
		10th	25th	50th	75th	90th		10th	25th	50th	75th	90th
All RDs	8621	$16.20	$18.75	$22.00	$26.79	$33.65	5319	$34,000	$38,900	$45,800	$56,000	$72,000
Number Supervised												
100+	203	$20.74	$26.92	$33.33	$39.90	$46.63	174	$44,200	$60,000	$74,500	$89,100	$108,000
50 - 99	290	$19.23	$23.08	$28.25	$33.51	$38.92	244	$42,300	$49,900	$60,000	$70,900	$83,300
10 - 49	1399	$17.31	$20.00	$24.04	$28.85	$34.33	1077	$36,400	$42,000	$50,000	$60,000	$72,800
1 - 9	2327	$16.35	$18.75	$21.63	$26.44	$33.62	1551	$34,000	$38,500	$44,800	$54,000	$70,000
0	4377	$15.63	$18.00	$21.01	$25.00	$30.46	2264	$33,000	$36,800	$42,900	$51,000	$61,300

Note: Results not shown if fewer than 25 valid values; 10th and 90th percentiles not shown if fewer than 50 valid values.

Exhibit 3.14

RD Compensation by Budget Responsibility

		HOURLY WAGE						TOTAL CASH COMPENSATION (those employed full time, 1+ years)				
	# answering	10th	25th	50th	75th	90th	# answering	10th	25th	50th	75th	90th
		— — — — — — percentiles — — — — — —						— — — — — — percentiles — — — — — —				
All RDs	8621	$16.20	$18.75	$22.00	$26.79	$33.65	5319	$34,000	$38,900	$45,800	$56,000	$72,000
Budget Responsibility												
$1,000K+	653	$21.63	$25.13	$30.77	$36.56	$44.76	583	$46,600	$55,000	$66,100	$80,000	$102,600
$500K - $999K	299	$20.00	$22.72	$26.11	$31.25	$40.00	254	$42,000	$48,000	$55,000	$68,100	$89,300
$100K - $499K	743	$17.47	$20.00	$24.04	$28.85	$35.66	587	$36,300	$41,800	$50,000	$62,000	$78,000
< $100K	657	$15.67	$18.75	$22.60	$28.44	$35.73	355	$33,900	$39,600	$47,000	$61,000	$77,400
does not apply	6090	$15.85	$18.10	$21.00	$25.00	$30.00	3432	$33,000	$37,000	$42,500	$50,000	$59,000

Note: Results not shown if fewer than 25 valid values; 10th and 90th percentiles not shown if fewer than 50 valid values.

Exhibit 3.15

RD Compensation by Location (Census Division)

		HOURLY WAGE						TOTAL CASH COMPENSATION (those employed full time, 1+ years)				
	# answering	10th	25th	50th	75th	90th	# answering	10th	25th	50th	75th	90th
		— — — — — — percentiles — — — — — —						— — — — — — percentiles — — — — — —				
All RDs	8621	$16.20	$18.75	$22.00	$26.79	$33.65	5319	$34,000	$38,900	$45,800	$56,000	$72,000
Employment Location (Census Division)												
New England	578	$17.30	$20.00	$23.75	$29.58	$36.70	300	$36,000	$40,800	$49,400	$60,000	$75,000
Middle Atlantic	1187	$16.67	$19.23	$23.00	$28.37	$35.71	771	$34,600	$39,600	$45,200	$55,300	$73,000
East North Central	1616	$16.32	$18.38	$21.00	$25.00	$31.29	954	$34,500	$38,200	$44,100	$53,500	$68,500
West North Central	839	$15.38	$17.31	$20.40	$25.00	$31.97	487	$32,200	$36,500	$43,700	$52,000	$68,600
South Atlantic	1445	$15.86	$18.27	$21.59	$25.96	$33.17	962	$33,000	$37,700	$45,000	$54,000	$69,000
East South Central	492	$15.38	$17.32	$20.19	$24.67	$31.45	336	$31,600	$35,000	$41,600	$52,400	$65,900
West South Central	766	$15.77	$17.79	$21.25	$25.96	$33.09	511	$32,800	$37,000	$44,000	$53,300	$69,600
Mountain	500	$15.88	$18.27	$20.99	$25.18	$32.69	288	$34,300	$38,100	$45,300	$55,000	$70,000
Pacific	1186	$19.21	$21.63	$25.00	$29.43	$35.86	702	$40,500	$45,700	$53,200	$65,000	$79,000

Note: Results not shown if fewer than 25 valid values; 10th and 90th percentiles not shown if fewer than 50 valid values.

Exhibit 3.16

RD Compensation by Location (State)

| | HOURLY WAGE | | | | | | TOTAL CASH COMPENSATION (those employed full time, 1+ years) | | | | | |
	# answering	10th	25th	50th	75th	90th	# answering	10th	25th	50th	75th	90th
All RDs	8621	$16.20	$18.75	$22.00	$26.79	$33.65	5319	$34,000	$38,900	$45,800	$56,000	$72,000
Employment Location (State)												
AK	14						7					
AL	119	$15.38	$17.55	$20.19	$24.52	$31.30	77	$31,100	$35,300	$41,600	$53,100	$66,000
AR	76	$14.94	$17.31	$20.89	$24.94	$30.89	49		$35,500	$45,000	$50,800	
AZ	123	$16.35	$18.03	$21.62	$26.34	$33.80	74	$34,200	$38,000	$45,800	$57,900	$80,000
CA	834	$19.23	$22.12	$25.39	$30.21	$36.78	505	$41,000	$47,100	$55,200	$67,000	$80,400
CO	129	$16.49	$19.23	$21.15	$24.88	$31.25	64	$35,800	$39,100	$45,200	$55,000	$70,000
CT	118	$19.23	$21.15	$25.93	$30.83	$35.10	62	$39,300	$45,600	$52,700	$63,300	$76,100
DC	45		$19.05	$26.92	$32.50		35		$37,700	$58,000	$68,000	
DE, MD	222	$18.39	$20.19	$24.04	$29.16	$36.06	138	$37,000	$43,300	$50,300	$60,500	$77,600
FL	371	$16.03	$18.27	$21.54	$25.64	$33.09	254	$33,300	$38,000	$45,000	$54,100	$68,800
GA	201	$16.32	$18.12	$21.63	$26.19	$33.65	130	$34,000	$38,000	$45,000	$54,000	$73,900
HI	42		$21.51	$23.92	$29.48		34		$45,000	$49,800	$61,200	
IA	149	$15.38	$16.92	$20.31	$25.00	$29.73	87	$32,900	$35,200	$43,000	$52,000	$61,900
ID, MT, WY	96	$14.42	$16.42	$19.37	$22.84	$28.90	58	$32,100	$38,000	$43,900	$48,400	$57,300
IL	405	$15.97	$18.75	$21.63	$27.15	$35.17	249	$34,800	$39,500	$45,900	$58,800	$80,500
IN	198	$15.14	$17.75	$20.14	$22.88	$28.85	132	$32,000	$36,900	$42,100	$47,000	$57,900
KS	102	$15.53	$17.31	$19.23	$23.49	$30.88	47		$34,400	$38,500	$47,000	
KY	121	$15.00	$17.15	$20.43	$24.04	$28.63	74	$31,500	$35,000	$42,300	$53,000	$65,600
LA	128	$14.89	$16.57	$19.23	$24.08	$30.33	83	$31,000	$34,000	$39,500	$50,000	$57,500
MA	281	$16.86	$19.71	$24.04	$30.85	$39.43	147	$35,000	$39,600	$49,200	$61,800	$77,400
MD, DE	222	$18.39	$20.19	$24.04	$29.16	$36.06	138	$37,000	$43,300	$50,300	$60,500	$77,600
ME, NH, VT	136	$16.71	$19.23	$21.40	$24.55	$31.92	66	$36,000	$40,000	$45,800	$51,700	$61,400
MI	292	$16.65	$18.27	$20.84	$25.00	$29.02	167	$34,800	$37,800	$42,000	$50,300	$61,200
MN	233	$16.41	$19.22	$22.12	$26.53	$35.58	144	$34,400	$40,000	$47,100	$56,000	$79,000
MO	202	$14.42	$16.83	$19.74	$23.73	$29.40	123	$31,500	$35,000	$41,600	$52,000	$65,100
MS	79	$15.38	$16.83	$19.23	$24.04	$32.29	59	$31,800	$33,700	$40,000	$47,800	$62,000
MT, ID, WY	96	$14.42	$16.42	$19.37	$22.84	$28.90	58	$32,100	$38,000	$43,900	$48,400	$57,300
NC	253	$15.60	$17.01	$20.01	$24.54	$29.11	166	$32,500	$35,500	$41,600	$51,400	$60,000
ND, SD	77	$14.33	$15.74	$19.90	$23.78	$30.05	36		$34,000	$40,900	$50,700	
NE	76	$14.86	$17.67	$20.27	$24.94	$31.70	50	$29,900	$36,700	$43,000	$48,900	$76,100
NH, ME, VT	136	$16.71	$19.23	$21.40	$24.55	$31.92	66	$36,000	$40,000	$45,800	$51,700	$61,400
NJ	227	$18.69	$21.15	$25.64	$29.67	$36.97	150	$38,300	$43,000	$51,300	$61,700	$82,400
NM	38		$18.63	$20.99	$22.93		21					
NV	46		$20.19	$24.04	$28.95		35		$47,000	$50,500	$62,000	
NY	551	$17.38	$20.19	$23.69	$29.56	$37.50	368	$35,000	$40,000	$47,100	$57,000	$74,900
OH	452	$16.00	$18.27	$20.80	$25.00	$31.11	263	$33,900	$38,000	$43,700	$52,000	$65,400
OK	79	$14.28	$17.28	$19.71	$24.04	$28.85	53	$31,400	$35,900	$41,000	$50,000	$59,500
OR	89	$17.79	$20.19	$23.08	$26.82	$30.00	46		$43,900	$48,300	$57,500	
PA	409	$15.38	$17.73	$20.19	$25.00	$30.29	253	$32,400	$37,000	$42,000	$51,300	$65,000
PR	28	$11.20	$12.42	$15.52	$21.03	$26.45	26	$23,200	$25,900	$32,900	$45,600	$62,100

Exhibit 3.16 (continued)

RD Compensation by Location (State)

| | # answering | HOURLY WAGE | | | | | # answering | TOTAL CASH COMPENSATION (those employed full time, 1+ years) | | | | |
		10th	25th	50th	75th	90th		10th	25th	50th	75th	90th
All RDs	8621	$16.20	$18.75	$22.00	$26.79	$33.65	5319	$34,000	$38,900	$45,800	$56,000	$72,000
Employment Location (State)												
RI	43		$23.00	$25.00	$31.25		25		$45,800	$52,000	$61,300	
SC	76	$15.59	$18.51	$21.63	$24.29	$30.00	53	$32,000	$35,500	$45,000	$50,300	$58,500
SD, ND	77	$14.33	$15.74	$19.90	$23.78	$30.05	36		$34,000	$40,900	$50,700	
TN	173	$15.15	$17.79	$20.51	$25.61	$32.38	126	$31,200	$36,300	$41,800	$54,200	$66,200
TX	483	$16.55	$18.73	$22.00	$27.00	$35.06	326	$34,500	$38,800	$45,200	$56,100	$78,100
UT	68	$15.57	$17.36	$20.67	$28.51	$33.66	36		$35,000	$44,000	$56,500	
VA	197	$15.56	$18.27	$20.83	$25.00	$30.53	126	$32,700	$37,400	$43,300	$51,400	$61,400
VT, ME, NH	136	$16.71	$19.23	$21.40	$24.55	$31.92	66	$36,000	$40,000	$45,800	$51,700	$61,400
WA	205	$17.11	$20.43	$23.96	$26.86	$33.65	108	$39,400	$43,300	$50,000	$58,400	$75,000
WI	269	$17.20	$19.17	$21.25	$24.72	$30.30	143	$36,000	$40,000	$45,600	$54,800	$69,400
WV	52	$15.13	$17.46	$20.51	$25.00	$28.93	34		$37,600	$42,500	$52,600	
WY, ID, MT	96	$14.42	$16.42	$19.37	$22.84	$28.90	58	$32,100	$38,000	$43,900	$48,400	$57,300

Note: Results not shown if fewer than 25 valid values; 10th and 90th percentiles not shown if fewer than 50 valid values.

Exhibit 3.17

RD Compensation by Location (Metro Area)

	# answering	HOURLY WAGE					# answering	TOTAL CASH COMPENSATION (those employed full time, 1+ years)				
		10th	25th	50th	75th	90th		10th	25th	50th	75th	90th
All RDs	8621	$16.20	$18.75	$22.00	$26.79	$33.65	5319	$34,000	$38,900	$45,800	$56,000	$72,000
Employment Location (Metropolitan Area)												
Albany-Schenectady-Troy, NY	46		$19.64	$27.75	$32.39		32		$38,900	$58,000	$70,700	
Atlanta, GA	120	$16.36	$19.05	$21.80	$28.89	$34.96	74	$34,100	$38,000	$45,900	$57,800	$77,800
Austin-San Marcos, TX	38		$17.41	$20.00	$26.90		21					
Baltimore, MD	112	$17.62	$20.00	$23.16	$26.88	$33.65	69	$36,500	$41,800	$48,400	$56,300	$70,000
Birmingham, AL	36		$16.17	$19.23	$24.04		25		$32,100	$36,000	$51,500	
Boston, MA-NH	167	$17.05	$19.79	$25.00	$32.00	$40.17	93	$35,100	$40,400	$50,000	$66,900	$80,000
Buffalo-Niagara Falls, NY	41		$18.22	$21.63	$24.45		29		$38,000	$45,000	$50,000	
Charlotte-Gastonia-Rock Hill, NC-SC	42		$19.69	$22.13	$25.50		25		$40,700	$47,000	$54,800	
Chicago, IL	293	$16.73	$19.23	$22.40	$27.94	$35.87	182	$36,500	$40,000	$46,000	$60,000	$84,400
Cincinnati, OH-KY-IN	78	$16.28	$19.98	$22.21	$26.50	$32.77	42		$41,900	$48,000	$55,600	
Cleveland-Lorain-Elyria, OH	91	$16.70	$18.50	$20.46	$25.64	$31.89	58	$34,700	$38,200	$42,900	$53,200	$65,000
Columbus, OH	90	$15.48	$19.08	$22.12	$26.71	$37.07	56	$33,700	$39,300	$46,000	$55,000	$91,100
Dallas, TX	101	$16.42	$18.51	$21.68	$26.49	$35.87	72	$35,100	$38,800	$45,900	$58,700	$88,100
Dayton-Springfield, OH	39		$18.37	$20.83	$24.13		18					
Denver, CO	61	$16.98	$19.23	$21.63	$25.60	$33.41	36		$42,000	$46,100	$59,100	
Detroit, MI	108	$16.83	$18.60	$20.35	$25.00	$28.92	65	$35,000	$38,200	$41,800	$50,900	$62,800
Fort Lauderdale, FL	31		$20.00	$23.00	$25.64		16					
Fort Worth-Arlington, TX	50	$17.67	$19.93	$23.32	$31.81	$43.92	33		$40,200	$47,100	$67,500	
Grand Rapids-Muskegon-Holland, MI	42		$16.34	$19.29	$22.82		24					
Greensboro-Winston-Salem-High Point, NC	44		$17.05	$19.83	$23.97		33		$35,100	$41,200	$50,400	
Hartford, CT	57	$16.73	$20.92	$26.00	$30.64	$35.33	28		$44,900	$51,700	$63,000	
Houston, TX	114	$16.85	$18.44	$22.82	$26.81	$32.84	86	$35,000	$37,000	$45,500	$55,500	$75,500
Indianapolis, IN	71	$14.42	$17.09	$19.26	$22.60	$27.83	50	$30,200	$36,200	$41,300	$47,000	$58,300
Kansas City, MO-KS	68	$15.08	$16.87	$19.18	$24.04	$28.92	39		$34,600	$39,500	$54,600	
Little Rock-North Little Rock, AR	40		$16.95	$22.96	$26.24		26		$35,600	$45,300	$54,900	
Los Angeles-Long Beach, CA	197	$19.95	$22.45	$25.00	$31.25	$38.46	130	$41,000	$47,400	$54,100	$72,100	$93,900
Louisville, KY-IN	47		$15.87	$19.00	$22.81		31		$32,800	$39,500	$50,000	
Madison, WI	36		$19.25	$21.54	$24.67		22					
Miami, FL	45		$19.23	$25.00	$28.85		31		$38,600	$51,400	$62,000	
Middlesex-Somerset-Hunterdon, NJ	35		$21.33	$25.29	$29.33		21					
Milwaukee-Waukesha, WI	83	$17.13	$18.49	$21.62	$26.59	$33.56	44		$40,100	$49,400	$63,800	
Minneapolis-St. Paul, MN-WI	141	$16.83	$19.23	$22.60	$26.92	$37.27	94	$35,700	$41,200	$48,300	$58,000	$89,700
Nashville, TN	49		$17.00	$21.15	$25.06		37		$37,800	$44,800	$57,200	
Nassau-Suffolk, NY	86	$19.23	$21.20	$23.94	$28.85	$42.64	47		$43,000	$49,000	$58,000	
New Orleans, LA	47		$16.83	$19.23	$25.00		36		$33,500	$39,800	$50,800	

Exhibit 3.17 (continued)

RD Compensation by Location (Metro Area)

	# answering	HOURLY WAGE percentiles					# answering	TOTAL CASH COMPENSATION (those employed full time, 1+ years) percentiles				
		10th	25th	50th	75th	90th		10th	25th	50th	75th	90th
All RDs	8621	$16.20	$18.75	$22.00	$26.79	$33.65	5319	$34,000	$38,900	$45,800	$56,000	$72,000
Employment Location (Metropolitan Area)												
New York, NY	224	$19.23	$21.30	$24.86	$31.23	$39.19	163	$38,000	$42,000	$49,000	$60,000	$72,000
Newark, NJ	73	$19.08	$21.88	$26.62	$30.50	$41.91	49		$43,200	$54,500	$62,700	
Norfolk-Virginia Beach-Newport News, VA-NC	45		$17.81	$20.67	$22.84		29		$36,000	$43,200	$47,500	
Oakland, CA	67	$22.31	$24.41	$28.00	$31.25	$39.52	45		$53,600	$60,300	$72,000	
Oklahoma City, OK	30		$16.76	$19.95	$23.43		22					
Omaha, NE-IA	33		$17.97	$20.19	$21.63		26		$36,700	$42,400	$49,000	
Orange County, CA	65	$19.46	$22.33	$26.11	$31.32	$42.00	37		$50,000	$58,300	$67,500	
Orlando, FL	37		$16.18	$18.59	$22.23		27		$34,300	$36,700	$48,500	
Philadelphia, PA-NJ	155	$17.31	$19.25	$22.73	$26.44	$31.57	99	$36,000	$40,000	$45,000	$54,200	$70,000
Phoenix-Mesa, AZ	81	$16.35	$18.25	$21.63	$27.65	$33.59	50	$34,000	$37,700	$43,300	$58,500	$80,000
Pittsburgh, PA	77	$14.62	$16.36	$19.23	$25.00	$29.28	49		$37,000	$41,000	$54,300	
Portland-Vancouver, OR-WA	63	$18.33	$20.19	$23.12	$27.26	$30.82	34		$43,500	$49,400	$57,500	
Providence-Fall River-Warwick, RI-MA	42		$22.66	$25.00	$31.37		23					
Raleigh-Durham-Chapel Hill, NC	61	$15.90	$18.27	$21.03	$25.44	$30.89	32		$37,800	$45,500	$53,000	
Richmond-Petersburg, VA	46		$18.21	$21.24	$25.00		29		$37,700	$44,000	$50,500	
Riverside-San Bernardino, CA	62	$18.26	$21.15	$24.52	$28.06	$35.05	46		$43,800	$52,000	$61,100	
Rochester, NY	43		$16.35	$19.47	$27.69		28		$33,200	$37,000	$49,200	
Sacramento, CA	56	$19.90	$23.56	$27.57	$32.09	$40.38	31		$51,000	$57,100	$69,000	
St. Louis, MO-IL	100	$13.95	$16.83	$19.99	$23.26	$28.85	60	$30,200	$35,400	$44,200	$54,800	$69,100
Salt Lake City-Ogden, UT	41		$17.95	$20.67	$29.81		23					
San Antonio, TX	33		$19.98	$23.00	$31.01		18					
San Diego, CA	84	$17.91	$20.05	$22.56	$28.80	$34.33	55	$35,700	$41,200	$50,300	$61,100	$81,000
San Francisco, CA	55	$20.52	$24.01	$27.24	$31.41	$38.50	35		$50,000	$57,000	$65,000	
San Jose, CA	48		$25.40	$28.75	$32.70		22					
Seattle-Bellevue-Everett, WA	86	$17.16	$20.63	$24.04	$27.92	$34.62	47		$42,500	$53,000	$69,400	
Tampa-St. Petersburg-Clearwater, FL	70	$15.89	$19.11	$23.05	$26.77	$33.84	51	$34,500	$39,100	$49,500	$59,800	$75,800
Washington, DC-MD-VA-WV	165	$16.83	$20.17	$25.00	$32.53	$40.65	114	$35,000	$40,600	$53,000	$69,300	$85,400
West Palm Beach-Boca Raton, FL	36		$19.57	$23.95	$27.88		25		$36,800	$50,000	$53,000	

Note: Results not shown if fewer than 25 valid values; 10th and 90th percentiles not shown if fewer than 50 valid values.

4. RD Salary Calculation Worksheet

Notes

On the following page you'll find an easy-to-use alternative for better understanding RD compensation — a Salary Calculation Worksheet.

As demonstrated by tables in the preceding section, numerous factors influence compensation levels. Tabular presentation, however, quickly exhausts even a large database such as this one when the joint effects of multiple factors are considered simultaneously.

For this reason, a second perspective on RD compensation is offered: a Salary Calculation Worksheet based on a multiple regression statistical model that attempts to predict compensation by accounting for the effects of 13 influential variables at the same time. In principle, this model allows estimation of compensation for thousands of possible combinations of the predictors.

Statistically speaking, the model is moderately powerful: it explains 54% of the variation in salary (adjusted R Square = 0.535), and is significant by the F test at $p < 0.0005$. Most predictors included in the model are significant by the t test at $p < 0.05$.

The model's predictive ability varies; predictions will tend to be most accurate for salary values in the middle of the range. The standard error of the predicted value averages $0.34, although it ranges from $0.18 to $0.96.

The statistical conclusions reached through this model must be interpreted carefully. Although a model explaining more than half of the variation in compensation may be described as "moderately powerful," it still leaves nearly half of the variation unexplained. It is certain that other variables not captured through this survey also have an effect on salary levels: individual job performance, for example. To the extent that this model does not include all the major determinants of compensation, it must be interpreted cautiously.

RD Salary Calculation Worksheet

This salary calculation worksheet is based on a statistical model developed with data from 5,470 full-time RDs with less than 50 years of experience and an hourly wage in the range of $11.54 to $51.33 (roughly $24,000 to $107,000 annualized). The model provides moderately powerful predictive accuracy within relatively broad ranges — offering a rough idea of what professionals with similar characteristics and in similar situations earn, on average. It also provides a sense of the relative importance of each factor in predicting salaries. Because other factors not included in the model are known to influence salary (for example, individual job performance), the model is not appropriately used as an absolute guideline for any single individual's situation.

STEP 1:
Find initial wage estimate based on the number of years since initial registration as an RD, and fill in at right. (For odd years, use the average of the two surrounding even years.)

Years Since Registration	Initial Wage Estimate
0	$18.36
2	$19.17
4	$19.93
6	$20.61
8	$21.23
10	$21.79
12	$22.28
14	$22.71
16	$23.07
18	$23.37
20	$23.61
22	$23.77
24	$23.88
26	$23.92
28	$23.89
30	$23.80
32	$23.65
34	$23.43
36	$23.15
38	$22.80
40	$22.38
42	$21.91
44	$21.36
46	$20.76
48	$20.09
50	$19.35

STEP 2:
Fill in other values as directed, based on the particular situation of interest.

STEP 3:
Sum all values together to calculate estimated hourly wage.

INITIAL WAGE ESTIMATE FROM STEP 1:　　　　　　　　　　　　　　$_____ / hr

Prior Experience
For each year of dietetics experience *prior* to becoming registered, add $0.05 x # of years 　　+ $_____

Education
If highest degree held is a master's degree, add $1.08
If highest degree held is a doctorate, add $5.79　　　　　　　　　　+ $_____

Credentials
If state licensed, **subtract** $0.49　　　　　　　　　　　　　　　- $_____
If hold one or more specialty certifications, add $0.52　　　　　　　+ $_____

Employer
If self-employed, add $4.51　　　　　　　　　　　　　　　　　　+ $_____
If employed by a nonprofit organization, **subtract** $1.06　　　　　　- $_____

If employer employs 500 to 999 people at all locations, add $0.71
If employer employs 1000+ people at all locations, add $1.53　　　　+ $_____

Practice Area
Add or subtract the indicated amount if position is in one of these practice areas:　　$_____

Clinical Nutrition — Acute Care/Inpatient	- $3.29
Clinical Nutrition — Ambulatory Care	- $2.59
Clinical Nutrition — Long Term Care	- $2.48
Community	- $3.39
Food and Nutrition Management	- $2.15
Consultation and Business	+ $0.70
Education and Research	- $1.28

Responsibility Level (choose one)
If an owner or partner, add $0.34
If an executive, add $4.79
If a director or manager, add $1.36
If a supervisor or coordinator, add $0.33　　　　　　　　　　　　+ $_____

For each person directly or indirectly supervised up to 100, add $0.03 x # supervised　　+ $_____

For each $100,000 of budget managed up to $1 million, add $0.04 x budget ($000,000)　　+ $_____

For each year in this position, add $0.07 x # of years in position　　+ $_____

Location
Add or subtract the indicated amount if location is in one of these Census Divisions:　　$_____

New England	+ $1.44
Middle Atlantic	+ $1.32
West North Central	- $0.94
East South Central	- $0.97
West South Central	- $0.44
Pacific	+ $2.89

STEP 3: Sum all entries in the righthand column to reach FINAL wage estimate: = $_____ / hr

5. DTR Compensation

Notes

Tables in this section report compensation for the 1,397 Dietetic Technicians, Registered (DTRs) who provided complete hour and compensation information. Results are broken out by a number of factors to demonstrate the relative effects of qualifications, experience, and employment situation in determining compensation levels.

Note that all factors are based on respondent self-reports and are thus subject to some variation in how terms were understood.

Two measures are reported: *hourly wage* and *total cash compensation*.

In accordance with Bureau of Labor Statistics practice, hourly wage may be converted to an annualized salary by multiplying the wage by 40 hours per week and 52 weeks per year.

Total cash compensation is reported only for practitioners employed or self-employed in the position full time for at least 1 year, and includes sources of compensation beyond salary/wage, such as bonuses, commissions, on-call pay, etc. For some workers, such as consultants, salespeople, and executives, a significant part of their compensation can come from sources other than salary. For such individuals, total cash compensation provides a more accurate picture of compensation than wages alone.

In addition to the number of individuals answering, 5 percentile values are reported for each measure: 10% of practitioners earn less than the 10th percentile, 25% earn less than the 25th percentile, and so on. All percentiles are suppressed if there are fewer than 25 valid responses; the 10th and 90th percentiles are suppressed if there are fewer than 50 valid responses.

Compensation by location is reported in terms of the nine standard Census Divisions:

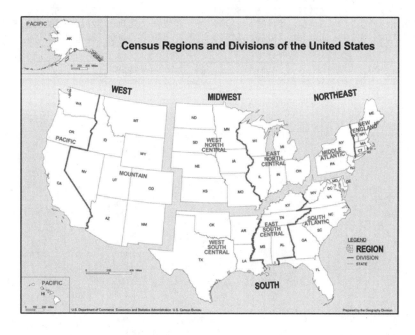

Exhibit 5.1

DTR Compensation by Years in Field

	# answering	HOURLY WAGE					# answering	TOTAL CASH COMPENSATION (those employed full time, 1+ years)				
		10th	25th	50th	75th	90th		10th	25th	50th	75th	90th
All DTRs	1397	$11.31	$12.82	$14.74	$16.97	$20.19	938	$23,900	$27,000	$31,000	$36,300	$43,100
Years In Field												
20+ years	336	$12.50	$14.01	$15.87	$18.56	$21.84	261	$26,100	$30,000	$33,800	$40,500	$49,800
10 - 19 years	483	$11.67	$13.46	$15.09	$17.31	$20.50	313	$25,000	$28,000	$31,500	$37,000	$44,000
5 - 9 years	353	$10.98	$12.02	$14.26	$16.25	$19.23	234	$22,300	$25,000	$29,900	$34,100	$40,000
< 5 years	222	$10.61	$11.54	$12.93	$14.58	$16.59	128	$21,900	$24,100	$27,400	$31,900	$35,400

Note: Results not shown if fewer than 25 valid values; 10th and 90th percentiles not shown if fewer than 50 valid values.

Exhibit 5.2

DTR Compensation by Years in Position

	# answering	HOURLY WAGE					# answering	TOTAL CASH COMPENSATION (those employed full time, 1+ years)				
		10th	25th	50th	75th	90th		10th	25th	50th	75th	90th
All DTRs	1397	$11.31	$12.82	$14.74	$16.97	$20.19	938	$23,900	$27,000	$31,000	$36,300	$43,100
Years In Position												
10+ years	479	$12.02	$13.78	$15.39	$18.18	$21.63	358	$25,000	$28,500	$32,000	$39,000	$46,200
5 - 9 years	359	$11.19	$12.75	$14.64	$16.92	$19.44	241	$23,000	$27,000	$30,500	$36,000	$41,400
< 5 years	558	$11.00	$12.02	$14.18	$16.13	$19.23	339	$23,000	$26,000	$30,000	$34,500	$42,000

Note: Results not shown if fewer than 25 valid values; 10th and 90th percentiles not shown if fewer than 50 valid values.

Exhibit 5.3

DTR Compensation by Education

	# answering	HOURLY WAGE					# answering	TOTAL CASH COMPENSATION (those employed full time, 1+ years)				
		10th	25th	50th	75th	90th		10th	25th	50th	75th	90th
All DTRs	1397	$11.31	$12.82	$14.74	$16.97	$20.19	938	$23,900	$27,000	$31,000	$36,300	$43,100
Education (Highest Degree)												
master's degree	35		$14.42	$21.25	$26.92		22					
bachelor's degree	312	$11.54	$13.46	$15.38	$18.27	$21.95	210	$25,000	$28,600	$32,800	$39,000	$49,900
associate's degree	1048	$11.17	$12.50	$14.42	$16.67	$19.23	704	$23,000	$26,700	$30,000	$35,000	$41,600

Note: Results not shown if fewer than 25 valid values; 10th and 90th percentiles not shown if fewer than 50 valid values.

Exhibit 5.4

DTR Compensation by Education and Years in Field

	# answering	HOURLY WAGE					# answering	TOTAL CASH COMPENSATION (those employed full time, 1+ years)				
		10th	25th	50th	75th	90th		10th	25th	50th	75th	90th
All DTRs	1397	$11.31	$12.82	$14.74	$16.97	$20.19	938	$23,900	$27,000	$31,000	$36,300	$43,100
bachelor's degree	312	$11.54	$13.46	$15.38	$18.27	$21.95	210	$25,000	$28,600	$32,800	$39,000	$49,900
20+ years	85	$13.55	$14.56	$16.83	$19.71	$23.43	64	$30,000	$32,000	$36,900	$42,100	$53,100
10 - 19 years	122	$12.05	$13.78	$15.75	$18.63	$22.81	80	$26,900	$29,000	$33,000	$39,000	$49,700
5 - 9 years	66	$11.06	$12.40	$14.26	$18.31	$21.30	41		$25,700	$30,000	$38,200	
< 5 years	38		$11.95	$14.09	$15.12		25		$24,400	$28,000	$32,000	
associate's degree	1048	$11.17	$12.50	$14.42	$16.67	$19.23	704	$23,000	$26,700	$30,000	$35,000	$41,600
20+ years	245	$12.02	$13.91	$15.48	$18.10	$21.41	192	$25,700	$28,800	$32,100	$40,000	$45,900
10 - 19 years	344	$11.57	$13.46	$14.98	$16.83	$19.23	222	$24,000	$28,000	$30,600	$35,100	$40,800
5 - 9 years	277	$10.58	$12.02	$14.18	$15.88	$18.27	188	$22,000	$25,000	$29,900	$33,800	$40,000
< 5 years	181	$10.58	$11.54	$12.82	$14.42	$16.78	101	$22,000	$24,300	$27,400	$31,200	$34,900

Note: Results not shown if fewer than 25 valid values; 10th and 90th percentiles not shown if fewer than 50 valid values.

Exhibit 5.5

DTR Compensation by Credentials Held

| | # answering | HOURLY WAGE | | | | | # answering | TOTAL CASH COMPENSATION (those employed full time, 1+ years) | | | | |
| | | percentiles | | | | | | percentiles | | | | |
		10th	25th	50th	75th	90th		10th	25th	50th	75th	90th
All DTRs	1397	$11.31	$12.82	$14.74	$16.97	$20.19	938	$23,900	$27,000	$31,000	$36,300	$43,100
Credentials Held												
state license	83	$11.61	$13.46	$15.60	$18.46	$22.98	52	$25,000	$28,300	$33,200	$40,000	$51,600
no state license	1314	$11.29	$12.82	$14.68	$16.83	$20.19	886	$23,800	$27,000	$30,800	$36,000	$43,000
specialty certification(s)	79	$11.41	$13.28	$15.00	$18.75	$22.00	58	$24,500	$27,500	$32,500	$40,200	$50,200
no specialty certification	1318	$11.29	$12.82	$14.71	$16.87	$20.19	880	$23,800	$27,000	$30,800	$36,000	$43,000

Note: Results not shown if fewer than 25 valid values; 10th and 90th percentiles not shown if fewer than 50 valid values.

Exhibit 5.5

DTR Compensation by ADA Membership

| | # answering | HOURLY WAGE | | | | | # answering | TOTAL CASH COMPENSATION (those employed full time, 1+ years) | | | | |
| | | percentiles | | | | | | percentiles | | | | |
		10th	25th	50th	75th	90th		10th	25th	50th	75th	90th
All DTRs	1397	$11.31	$12.82	$14.74	$16.97	$20.19	938	$23,900	$27,000	$31,000	$36,300	$43,100
ADA Membership												
ADA member	769	$11.46	$12.98	$15.00	$17.79	$21.50	543	$24,000	$27,200	$31,600	$38,000	$45,900
not a member	628	$11.07	$12.51	$14.42	$16.35	$19.23	395	$23,000	$26,500	$30,000	$34,300	$40,800

Note: Results not shown if fewer than 25 valid values; 10th and 90th percentiles not shown if fewer than 50 valid values.

Exhibit 5.7

DTR Compensation by Practice Area

	# answering	HOURLY WAGE					# answering	TOTAL CASH COMPENSATION (those employed full time, 1+ years)				
		10th	25th	50th	75th	90th		10th	25th	50th	75th	90th
All DTRs	1397	$11.31	$12.82	$14.74	$16.97	$20.19	938	$23,900	$27,000	$31,000	$36,300	$43,100
Practice Area												
clinical nutrition — acute care/inpatient	561	$11.06	$12.50	$14.42	$15.87	$17.59	384	$23,000	$26,000	$30,000	$33,000	$37,200
clinical nutrition — ambulatory care	7						3					
clinical nutrition — long term care	285	$11.52	$12.71	$14.42	$16.46	$18.38	189	$24,000	$26,300	$30,000	$34,400	$38,500
community	139	$10.58	$12.02	$13.94	$15.87	$18.75	78	$21,200	$25,000	$28,300	$33,100	$38,000
food and nutrition management	291	$12.02	$14.42	$16.83	$20.19	$25.61	218	$27,000	$30,500	$36,200	$43,800	$55,100
consultation and business	30		$13.41	$17.47	$21.77		18					
education and research	16						8					

Note: Results not shown if fewer than 25 valid values; 10th and 90th percentiles not shown if fewer than 50 valid values.

Exhibit 5.8

DTR Compensation by Practice Area and Years in Field

		HOURLY WAGE						TOTAL CASH COMPENSATION (those employed full time, 1+ years)				
	# answering	10th	25th	50th	75th	90th	# answering	10th	25th	50th	75th	90th
All DTRs	1397	$11.31	$12.82	$14.74	$16.97	$20.19	938	$23,900	$27,000	$31,000	$36,300	$43,100
clinical nutrition — acute care/inpatient	561	$11.06	$12.50	$14.42	$15.87	$17.59	384	$23,000	$26,000	$30,000	$33,000	$37,200
20+ years	148	$12.50	$13.86	$15.38	$16.83	$19.14	110	$25,600	$28,500	$31,800	$35,000	$39,800
10 - 19 years	205	$11.39	$12.99	$14.54	$15.87	$17.69	136	$22,900	$27,000	$30,000	$33,200	$37,400
5 - 9 years	127	$10.57	$11.75	$13.46	$15.11	$17.26	88	$22,000	$24,000	$28,100	$31,000	$35,900
< 5 years	81	$10.60	$11.41	$12.24	$13.97	$15.94	50	$22,100	$24,000	$27,000	$30,400	$33,400
clinical nutrition — long term care	285	$11.52	$12.71	$14.42	$16.46	$18.38	189	$24,000	$26,300	$30,000	$34,400	$38,500
20+ years	55	$11.77	$13.85	$14.92	$17.79	$21.25	44		$28,500	$31,600	$37,900	
10 - 19 years	96	$11.86	$13.46	$14.97	$16.83	$18.51	60	$25,200	$28,000	$31,100	$35,800	$38,900
5 - 9 years	80	$11.54	$12.27	$13.68	$15.56	$17.98	53	$23,000	$25,000	$28,000	$31,800	$37,300
< 5 years	54	$10.47	$11.82	$13.48	$15.38	$17.30	32		$24,600	$27,200	$31,500	
community	139	$10.58	$12.02	$13.94	$15.87	$18.75	78	$21,200	$25,000	$28,300	$33,100	$38,000
20+ years	16						11					
10 - 19 years	41		$13.45	$15.03	$16.62		24					
5 - 9 years	47		$11.48	$13.38	$15.63		27		$23,900	$26,600	$32,500	
< 5 years	35		$11.54	$12.50	$13.99		16					
food and nutrition management	291	$12.02	$14.42	$16.83	$20.19	$25.61	218	$27,000	$30,500	$36,200	$43,800	$55,100
20+ years	92	$13.39	$15.59	$18.22	$21.60	$26.78	81	$29,200	$34,100	$41,000	$50,000	$65,000
10 - 19 years	101	$12.15	$14.71	$16.93	$20.30	$26.35	68	$26,900	$30,100	$36,200	$44,100	$58,700
5 - 9 years	64	$11.13	$13.48	$15.63	$19.23	$24.52	45		$30,000	$35,000	$41,200	
< 5 years	33		$12.62	$14.06	$15.85		23					

Note: Results not shown if fewer than 25 valid values; 10th and 90th percentiles not shown if fewer than 50 valid values.

Exhibit 5.9

DTR Compensation by Employment Setting

| | # answering | HOURLY WAGE | | | | | # answering | TOTAL CASH COMPENSATION (those employed full time, 1+ years) | | | | |
		10th	25th	50th	75th	90th		10th	25th	50th	75th	90th
		- - - - - - - percentiles - - - - - -						- - - - - - - percentiles - - - - - -				
All DTRs	1397	$11.31	$12.82	$14.74	$16.97	$20.19	938	$23,900	$27,000	$31,000	$36,300	$43,100
Employment Setting												
hospital	505	$11.05	$12.49	$14.42	$16.27	$19.23	352	$23,000	$26,100	$30,000	$34,400	$40,900
extended care facility	449	$11.54	$12.98	$14.90	$16.98	$19.23	318	$25,000	$27,500	$31,000	$36,600	$42,000
community or public health												
program	131	$10.17	$12.44	$13.90	$15.63	$17.96	74	$21,600	$26,000	$28,300	$32,100	$37,700
government agency	31		$14.90	$17.31	$21.63		28		$32,000	$36,500	$44,200	
school food service	48		$14.86	$18.22	$22.61		19					

Note: Results not shown if fewer than 25 valid values; 10th and 90th percentiles not shown if fewer than 50 valid values.

Exhibit 5.10

DTR Compensation by Employer Status

| | # answering | HOURLY WAGE | | | | | # answering | TOTAL CASH COMPENSATION (those employed full time, 1+ years) | | | | |
		10th	25th	50th	75th	90th		10th	25th	50th	75th	90th
		- - - - - - - percentiles - - - - - -						- - - - - - - percentiles - - - - - -				
All DTRs	1397	$11.31	$12.82	$14.74	$16.97	$20.19	938	$23,900	$27,000	$31,000	$36,300	$43,100
Employer Status												
self-employed	26		$12.37	$17.03	$26.41		9					
for-profit	446	$11.27	$12.50	$14.57	$16.94	$20.19	314	$24,000	$27,000	$30,800	$36,800	$42,900
nonprofit												
(other than government)	669	$11.41	$12.82	$14.42	$16.83	$19.56	439	$23,000	$27,000	$30,500	$36,000	$43,000
government	223	$11.35	$13.46	$15.38	$18.03	$22.16	158	$24,000	$28,200	$32,000	$37,900	$45,000

Note: Results not shown if fewer than 25 valid values; 10th and 90th percentiles not shown if fewer than 50 valid values.

Exhibit 5.11

DTR Compensation by Size of Organization

	# answering	HOURLY WAGE					# answering	TOTAL CASH COMPENSATION (those employed full time, 1+ years)				
		percentiles						percentiles				
		10th	25th	50th	75th	90th		10th	25th	50th	75th	90th
All DTRs	1397	$11.31	$12.82	$14.74	$16.97	$20.19	938	$23,900	$27,000	$31,000	$36,300	$43,100
Size of Organization (Number Employed)												
1,000 or more	440	$11.47	$12.98	$15.00	$17.19	$20.19	312	$24,000	$27,400	$31,500	$37,000	$44,800
100 - 999	563	$11.50	$12.98	$14.90	$17.48	$20.19	390	$24,000	$27,000	$31,000	$37,400	$43,800
10 - 99	247	$10.58	$12.50	$14.42	$16.35	$19.29	159	$23,000	$26,700	$30,100	$34,200	$41,000
2 - 9	86	$10.03	$11.94	$14.16	$15.22	$18.18	53	$19,200	$24,000	$29,500	$32,000	$40,000
1 (self-employed)	21						6					

Note: Results not shown if fewer than 25 valid values; 10th and 90th percentiles not shown if fewer than 50 valid values.

Exhibit 5.12

DTR Compensation by Responsibility Level

	# answering	HOURLY WAGE					# answering	TOTAL CASH COMPENSATION (those employed full time, 1+ years)				
		percentiles						percentiles				
		10th	25th	50th	75th	90th		10th	25th	50th	75th	90th
All DTRs	1397	$11.31	$12.82	$14.74	$16.97	$20.19	938	$23,900	$27,000	$31,000	$36,300	$43,100
Responsibility Level												
owner or partner	14						5					
executive	5						4					
director or manager	295	$12.64	$14.74	$16.83	$20.19	$24.42	239	$27,000	$31,100	$37,000	$43,000	$54,500
supervisor or coordinator	339	$11.31	$12.82	$14.85	$16.99	$19.60	229	$24,000	$27,000	$30,600	$35,100	$42,000
other	733	$11.06	$12.30	$14.18	$15.87	$18.00	453	$22,900	$26,000	$29,300	$32,700	$37,000

Note: Results not shown if fewer than 25 valid values; 10th and 90th percentiles not shown if fewer than 50 valid values.

ADA 2002 Dietetics Compensation & Benefits Survey

Exhibit 5.13

DTR Compensation by Number Supervised

| | HOURLY WAGE | | | | | | TOTAL CASH COMPENSATION (those employed full time, 1+ years) | | | | | |
	# answering	10th	25th	50th	75th	90th	# answering	10th	25th	50th	75th	90th
		- - - - - - percentiles - - - - - -						- - - - - - percentiles - - - - - -				
All DTRs	1397	$11.31	$12.82	$14.74	$16.97	$20.19	938	$23,900	$27,000	$31,000	$36,300	$43,100
Number Supervised												
100+	20						16					
50 - 99	36		$15.69	$17.45	$24.76		30		$32,600	$40,800	$54,100	
10 - 49	422	$12.01	$13.57	$15.38	$18.27	$20.90	332	$25,100	$28,500	$32,800	$40,000	$45,000
1 - 9	243	$11.02	$12.88	$14.66	$16.83	$20.44	152	$23,700	$27,000	$30,600	$35,000	$43,100
0	668	$11.06	$12.30	$14.28	$15.87	$18.27	402	$22,400	$25,900	$29,500	$33,000	$37,800

Note: Results not shown if fewer than 25 valid values; 10th and 90th percentiles not shown if fewer than 50 valid values.

Exhibit 5.14

DTR Compensation by Budget Responsibility

| | HOURLY WAGE | | | | | | TOTAL CASH COMPENSATION (those employed full time, 1+ years) | | | | | |
	# answering	10th	25th	50th	75th	90th	# answering	10th	25th	50th	75th	90th
		- - - - - - percentiles - - - - - -						- - - - - - percentiles - - - - - -				
All DTRs	1397	$11.31	$12.82	$14.74	$16.97	$20.19	938	$23,900	$27,000	$31,000	$36,300	$43,100
Budget Responsibility												
$1,000K+	47		$16.83	$21.20	$26.20		41		$35,000	$45,000	$55,500	
$500K - $999K	42		$17.99	$20.09	$23.87		38		$37,300	$42,100	$52,100	
$100K - $499K	159	$12.88	$14.42	$16.35	$18.75	$20.67	121	$27,100	$30,300	$35,000	$41,100	$46,300
< $100K	90	$10.42	$12.02	$14.42	$16.48	$19.93	64	$24,000	$26,000	$31,200	$36,000	$42,000
does not apply	995	$11.06	$12.50	$14.42	$16.07	$18.75	631	$23,000	$26,000	$30,000	$33,400	$38,400

Note: Results not shown if fewer than 25 valid values; 10th and 90th percentiles not shown if fewer than 50 valid values.

Exhibit 5.15

DTR Compensation by Location (Census Division)

	HOURLY WAGE						**TOTAL CASH COMPENSATION** (those employed full time, 1+ years)					
	# answering	10th	25th	50th	75th	90th	# answering	10th	25th	50th	75th	90th
		- - - - - - - percentiles - - - - - - -						- - - - - - - percentiles - - - - - - -				
All DTRs	1397	$11.31	$12.82	$14.74	$16.97	$20.19	938	$23,900	$27,000	$31,000	$36,300	$43,100
Employment Location (Census Division)												
New England	119	$11.50	$13.46	$15.00	$17.00	$19.23	65	$25,000	$29,700	$31,900	$38,400	$43,800
Middle Atlantic	326	$11.43	$12.93	$14.59	$17.18	$21.54	222	$23,900	$27,000	$30,000	$36,000	$45,000
East North Central	400	$11.54	$12.73	$14.42	$16.19	$19.23	266	$24,000	$27,000	$30,100	$35,000	$42,200
West North Central	120	$11.26	$12.55	$14.50	$16.12	$19.23	78	$22,900	$27,100	$31,100	$35,000	$41,500
South Atlantic	183	$10.71	$12.50	$15.38	$18.27	$21.36	138	$23,000	$26,800	$32,900	$38,000	$43,000
East South Central	27		$12.02	$14.42	$16.83		23					
West South Central	52	$9.22	$10.68	$13.05	$15.89	$19.90	37		$24,000	$27,200	$32,900	
Mountain	34		$12.36	$14.20	$15.85		20					
Pacific	136	$12.01	$13.99	$15.93	$18.31	$23.07	89	$27,000	$30,000	$34,100	$38,400	$50,000

Note: Results not shown if fewer than 25 valid values; 10th and 90th percentiles not shown if fewer than 50 valid values.

Exhibit 5.16

DTR Compensation by Location (Selected States)

	HOURLY WAGE						TOTAL CASH COMPENSATION (those employed full time, 1+ years)					
	# answering	10th	25th	50th	75th	90th	# answering	10th	25th	50th	75th	90th
		------- percentiles -------						------- percentiles -------				
All DTRs	1397	$11.31	$12.82	$14.74	$16.97	$20.19	938	$23,900	$27,000	$31,000	$36,300	$43,100
Employment Location (State)												
CA	90	$12.17	$14.39	$16.35	$18.81	$23.77	68	$27,000	$30,000	$34,200	$39,000	$50,200
CT	34		$14.75	$16.56	$18.39		24					
DC, DE, MD	29		$13.74	$16.83	$19.71		24					
FL	101	$10.58	$12.30	$15.38	$18.23	$21.43	69	$22,000	$25,700	$33,300	$37,900	$42,000
IL, IN	58	$11.54	$13.07	$15.00	$17.36	$19.76	46		$27,100	$31,400	$37,700	
MA	27		$14.92	$16.18	$17.31		12					
ME, NH, VT	55	$11.02	$12.00	$14.00	$15.50	$17.88	28		$26,600	$30,000	$35,000	
MI	25		$13.46	$14.42	$16.71		19					
MN	59	$11.54	$13.30	$15.29	$16.83	$19.62	36		$29,600	$32,300	$37,000	
MO	33		$11.89	$14.42	$16.07		20					
NJ	33		$12.55	$15.00	$20.75		22					
NY	205	$11.63	$12.82	$14.71	$16.92	$20.04	137	$23,800	$26,000	$30,000	$34,000	$41,200
OH	229	$11.08	$12.59	$14.42	$16.14	$19.23	148	$23,000	$26,800	$30,000	$34,100	$42,100
OR, WA	43		$13.46	$15.26	$18.00		18					
PA	88	$11.05	$13.13	$14.42	$17.12	$23.08	63	$24,500	$27,500	$30,100	$37,800	$52,000
TX	26		$11.54	$13.46	$17.14		20					
VA	28		$12.03	$14.18	$16.83		25		$25,500	$30,000	$35,000	
WI	88	$11.54	$12.83	$14.42	$15.97	$20.05	53	$24,000	$27,000	$30,000	$34,200	$49,800

Note: Results not shown if fewer than 25 valid values; 10th and 90th percentiles not shown if fewer than 50 valid values.

6. DTR Salary Calculation Worksheet

Notes

On the following page you'll find an easy-to-use alternative for better understanding DTR compensation — a Salary Calculation Worksheet.

As demonstrated by tables in the preceding section, numerous factors influence compensation levels. Tabular presentation, however, quickly exhausts even a large database such as this one when the joint effects of multiple factors are considered simultaneously.

For this reason, a second perspective on DTR compensation is offered: a Salary Calculation Worksheet based on a multiple regression statistical model that attempts to predict compensation by accounting for the effects of 10 influential variables at the same time. In principle, this model allows estimation of compensation for thousands of possible combinations of the predictors.

Statistically speaking, the model is modestly powerful: it explains 42% of the variation in salary (adjusted R Square = 0.417), and is significant by the F test at $p < 0.0005$. Most predictors included in the model are significant by the t test at $p < 0.05$.

The model's predictive ability varies; predictions will tend to be most accurate for salary values in the middle of the range. The standard error of the predicted value averages $0.38, though it ranges from $0.19 to $1.32.

The statistical conclusions reached through this model must be interpreted carefully. While a model explaining somewhat less than half of the variation in compensation may be described as "modestly powerful," it still leaves more than half of the variation unexplained. It is certain that other variables not captured through this survey also have an effect on salary levels: individual job performance, for example. To the extent that this model does not include all the major determinants of compensation, it must be interpreted cautiously.

DTR Salary Calculation Worksheet

This salary calculation worksheet is based on a statistical model developed with data from 961 full-time DTRs with an hourly wage in the range of $8.31 to $32.26 (roughly $17,000 to $67,000 annualized). The model provides modestly powerful predictive accuracy within relatively broad ranges — offering a rough idea of what professionals with similar characteristics and in similar situations earn, on average. It also provides a sense of the relative importance of each factor in predicting salaries. Because other factors not included in the model are known to influence salary (for example, individual job performance), the model is not appropriately used as an absolute guideline for any single individual's situation.

STEP 1:
Find initial wage estimate based on the number of years since initial registration as a DTR, and fill in at right. (For odd years, use the average of the two surrounding even years.)

Years Since Registration	Initial Wage Estimate
0	$13.45
2	$13.73
4	$14.00
6	$14.27
8	$14.54
10	$14.81
12	$15.09
14	$15.36
16	$15.63
18	$15.90
20	$16.17
22	$16.45
24	$16.72
26	$16.99
28	$17.26
30	$17.53
32	$17.81
34	$18.08
36	$18.35
38	$18.62
40	$18.89
42	$19.17
44	$19.44
46	$19.71
48	$19.98
50	$20.25

STEP 2:
Fill in other values as directed, based on the particular situation of interest.

STEP 3:
Sum all values together to calculate estimated hourly wage.

INITIAL WAGE ESTIMATE FROM STEP 1: $_____ / hr

Prior Experience
For each year of dietetics experience *prior* to becoming registered, add $0.05 x # of years   + $_____

Education
If highest degree held is a bachelor's degree, add $0.90
If highest degree held is a master's degree, add $3.02   + $_____

Employer
If self-employed, add $4.08
If employed by government, add $1.28   + $_____

Add the indicated amount based on the number employed at all locations of your organization: + $_____
1 (self-employed)	$0.00
2 - 4	$0.01
5 - 9	$0.02
10 - 24	$0.04
25 - 49	$0.08
50 - 99	$0.16
100 - 249	$0.36
250 - 499	$0.64
500 - 999	$0.83
1000+	$0.70

Practice Area
Subtract the indicated amount if position is in one of these practice areas: - $_____
Clinical Nutrition — Acute Care/Inpatient	- $1.85
Clinical Nutrition — Long Term Care	- $1.98
Community	- $2.28
Food and Nutrition Management	- $0.99

Responsibility Level
If a director or manager, add $1.40   + $_____

For each person directly or indirectly supervised up to 100, add $0.02 x # supervised   + $_____

For each $100,000 of budget managed up to $1 million, add $0.04 x budget ($000,000)   + $_____

Location
Add or subtract the indicated amount if located in one of the following Census Divisions: $_____
West North Central	- $0.79
East South Central	- $1.30
West South Central	- $1.32
Pacific	+ $1.17

STEP 3: Sum all entries in the righthand column to reach FINAL wage estimate:	= $_____ / hr

7. Compensation by Position

Notes

Tables in this section report compensation by position.

Respondents were asked to match their job to one of 58 core position descriptions developed by the ADA, regardless of whether the position title was similar to their own. 95% of respondents selected one of the core positions; thus these data can be thought of as representing the vast majority of dietetics practice.

The brief description for each position is reproduced at the top of its table.

Sufficient responses were received to report at least minimal compensation data in all but four circumstances. A number of Clinical Dietitian, Specialist positions have been aggregated as Clinical Dietitian, Specialist — Other. Similarly, a number of Outpatient Dietitian, Specialist positions have been aggregated as Outpatient Dietitian, Specialist — Other. Finally, there were insufficient responses from Corrections Dietitians and Didactic Program Directors to report compensation statistics (however, those tables are included in the set for completeness).

For each position, results are broken out by a number of factors to demonstrate the relative effects on compensation: years in field, years in position, education, credentials held, type of employer, and responsibilities.

Note that all factors are based on respondent self-reports and are thus subject to some variation in how terms were understood.

Two measures are reported: *hourly wage* and *total cash compensation.*

In accordance with Bureau of Labor Statistics practice, hourly wage may be converted to an annualized salary by multiplying the wage by 40 hours per week and 52 weeks per year.

Total cash compensation is reported only for practitioners employed or self-employed in the position full time for at least 1 year, and includes sources of compensation beyond salary/wages, such as bonuses, commissions, on-call pay, etc. Total cash compensation provides a more accurate picture of compensation than wages alone for positions where a significant fraction of compensation does not come from salary (eg, consultants, salespeople, executives).

In addition to the number answering, 3 percentile values are reported for each measure: 25% of practitioners earn less than the 25th percentile, 50% earn less than the 50th percentile, and so on. Percentiles are suppressed if there are fewer than 25 valid responses.

Exhibit 7.1

Compensation: Dietetic Technician, Clinical

Conducts nutrition screening and routine assessments. Coordinates menu selections with diet order. Develops and implements nutrition care plans for assigned patients. Provides individualized or group nutrition education. Monitors quality and accuracy of food served to patients.

	HOURLY WAGE				**TOTAL CASH COMPENSATION** (those employed full time, 1+ years)			
	# answering	25th	50th	75th	# answering	25th	50th	75th
		-- percentiles --				-- percentiles --		
TOTAL	553	$12.45	$14.42	$15.87	380	$26,000	$30,000	$33,000
Years In Field								
20+ years	141	$13.80	$15.38	$16.83	106	$28,200	$31,400	$35,000
10 - 19 years	203	$12.98	$14.55	$15.90	137	$27,000	$30,000	$33,200
5 - 9 years	120	$11.70	$13.45	$15.09	82	$24,100	$28,000	$31,000
< 5 years	89	$11.45	$12.59	$14.42	55	$24,000	$27,000	$31,000
Years In Position								
10+ years	248	$13.46	$14.95	$16.40	181	$27,200	$30,200	$34,300
5 - 9 years	125	$12.02	$13.89	$15.44	84	$25,300	$29,200	$33,300
< 5 years	179	$11.80	$13.46	$14.90	115	$25,000	$28,200	$31,000
Education (Highest Degree)								
doctoral degree	1				1			
master's degree	7				5			
bachelor's degree	112	$12.99	$14.71	$16.83	76	$27,300	$31,000	$34,300
associate's degree	433	$12.02	$14.27	$15.63	298	$25,900	$29,400	$32,700
Credentials Held								
RD	15				11			
DTR	534	$12.42	$14.42	$15.87	367	$26,000	$30,000	$33,000
state license	30	$12.02	$15.07	$16.62	17			
specialty certification(s)	26	$12.74	$14.57	$16.62	19			
Employer								
self-employed	2				2			
for-profit	189	$12.02	$14.10	$15.63	125	$26,000	$29,400	$32,000
nonprofit (other than government)	290	$12.32	$14.22	$15.72	196	$25,100	$29,100	$33,000
government	55	$13.90	$15.87	$17.21	46	$30,000	$32,800	$35,300
Responsibilities								
director, manager or higher	34	$14.03	$15.87	$17.98	23			
supervise 1+ employees	192	$12.50	$14.42	$16.04	142	$27,000	$30,000	$33,500
supervise none	359	$12.44	$14.42	$15.87	236	$26,000	$30,000	$33,000
have budget responsibility	35	$12.50	$14.90	$17.31	28	$26,000	$31,100	$37,500
no budget responsibility	502	$12.21	$14.42	$15.87	342	$26,000	$30,000	$32,900

Note: Results not shown if fewer than 25 valid values.

Exhibit 7.2

Compensation: Clinical Dietitian

Performs comprehensive nutrition assessments. Develops and implements nutrition care plans. Provides medical nutrition therapy and nutrition education. May coordinate and supervise activities of DTRs and students.

	HOURLY WAGE				TOTAL CASH COMPENSATION (those employed full time, 1+ years)			
	# answering	-- percentiles -- 25th	50th	75th	# answering	-- percentiles -- 25th	50th	75th
TOTAL	1462	$17.03	$19.23	$22.00	924	$35,000	$39,900	$45,000
Years In Field								
20+ years	401	$19.23	$21.63	$24.08	239	$41,000	$45,000	$50,400
10 - 19 years	348	$18.51	$20.19	$22.96	179	$38,300	$41,900	$47,000
5 - 9 years	266	$16.83	$18.30	$20.55	162	$34,600	$38,000	$42,000
< 5 years	444	$15.46	$17.08	$19.00	342	$32,600	$35,900	$39,000
Years In Position								
10+ years	429	$19.23	$21.21	$24.04	266	$40,000	$45,000	$50,000
5 - 9 years	248	$17.45	$19.35	$22.10	149	$36,000	$40,000	$44,900
< 5 years	780	$16.30	$18.08	$20.19	509	$33,300	$37,000	$41,500
Education (Highest Degree)								
doctoral degree	5				3			
master's degree	464	$17.70	$19.99	$22.82	300	$36,400	$40,900	$46,600
bachelor's degree	974	$16.83	$19.23	$21.63	607	$35,000	$38,800	$44,300
associate's degree	16				13			
Credentials Held								
RD	1420	$17.25	$19.23	$22.04	896	$35,000	$40,000	$45,000
DTR	22				14			
state license	756	$16.83	$19.00	$21.34	476	$34,300	$38,300	$44,000
specialty certification(s)	145	$19.00	$20.67	$23.71	101	$39,000	$45,000	$50,200
Employer								
self-employed	25	$18.73	$27.00	$30.00	3			
for-profit	469	$16.53	$18.51	$20.65	295	$34,000	$38,000	$42,000
nonprofit (other than government)	825	$17.31	$19.23	$22.00	523	$35,500	$40,000	$45,000
government	115	$19.23	$23.08	$26.02	89	$38,000	$47,300	$54,000
Responsibilities								
director, manager or higher	144	$16.83	$19.68	$23.08	105	$35,000	$39,700	$45,000
supervise 1+ employees	640	$17.32	$19.67	$22.14	424	$36,000	$40,000	$45,600
supervise none	818	$16.83	$19.23	$21.63	498	$34,200	$38,800	$44,900
have budget responsibility	92	$17.08	$19.71	$22.32	67	$36,900	$41,000	$46,200
no budget responsibility	1350	$17.00	$19.23	$21.99	847	$35,000	$39,500	$45,000

Note: Results not shown if fewer than 25 valid values.

Exhibit 7.3

Compensation: Clinical Dietitian, Specialist — Cardiac

In addition to the duties described for the Clinical Dietitian, provides medical nutrition therapy for inpatients in a specialty area (devotes more than 50% of time to this specialty).

	HOURLY WAGE				TOTAL CASH COMPENSATION (those employed full time, 1+ years)			
	# answering	25th	-- percentiles -- 50th	75th	# answering	25th	-- percentiles -- 50th	75th
TOTAL	63	$17.31	$19.13	$20.19	49	$35,300	$39,500	$43,500
Years In Field								
20+ years	15				12			
10 - 19 years	17				11			
5 - 9 years	12				8			
< 5 years	19				18			
Years In Position								
10+ years	20				16			
5 - 9 years	10				7			
< 5 years	33	$15.90	$18.53	$19.43	26	$32,300	$36,300	$39,800
Education (Highest Degree)								
doctoral degree								
master's degree	21				12			
bachelor's degree	40	$17.60	$19.11	$20.96	36	$35,200	$39,100	$44,100
associate's degree	1							
Credentials Held								
RD	61	$17.37	$19.13	$20.19	48	$35,200	$39,300	$44,100
DTR	1							
state license	34	$17.19	$19.18	$20.45	25	$35,500	$39,800	$44,800
specialty certification(s)	7				5			
Employer								
self-employed								
for-profit	17				15			
nonprofit (other than government)	44	$17.38	$19.34	$21.23	32	$36,000	$40,400	$44,900
government	2				2			
Responsibilities								
director, manager or higher	2				2			
supervise 1+ employees	15				13			
supervise none	48	$16.83	$18.84	$20.93	36	$34,300	$38,800	$44,200
have budget responsibility	1				1			
no budget responsibility	62	$17.25	$19.06	$20.45	48	$35,200	$39,300	$44,100

Note: Results not shown if fewer than 25 valid values.

Exhibit 7.4

Compensation: Clinical Dietitian, Specialist — Diabetes

In addition to the duties described for the Clinical Dietitian, provides medical nutrition therapy for inpatients in a specialty area (devotes more than 50% of time to this specialty).

	HOURLY WAGE				TOTAL CASH COMPENSATION (those employed full time, 1+ years)			
	# answering	-- percentiles -- 25th	50th	75th	# answering	-- percentiles -- 25th	50th	75th
TOTAL	136	$18.30	$20.67	$24.04	76	$37,500	$42,100	$49,600
Years In Field								
20+ years	55	$20.05	$23.08	$25.00	30	$41,300	$48,200	$52,600
10 - 19 years	36	$20.21	$21.50	$24.10	16			
5 - 9 years	23				14			
< 5 years	22				16			
Years In Position								
10+ years	45	$20.19	$22.00	$25.00	26	$42,600	$46,900	$52,300
5 - 9 years	32	$18.17	$21.57	$26.88	18			
< 5 years	59	$17.07	$19.23	$22.79	32	$34,400	$38,000	$46,000
Education (Highest Degree)								
doctoral degree								
master's degree	65	$19.23	$20.83	$24.59	33	$39,100	$41,700	$51,300
bachelor's degree	70	$17.34	$20.46	$24.04	43	$35,400	$42,200	$49,000
associate's degree								
Credentials Held								
RD	136	$18.30	$20.67	$24.04	76	$37,500	$42,100	$49,600
DTR								
state license	73	$17.54	$20.41	$23.20	45	$35,700	$42,200	$50,000
specialty certification(s)	84	$19.87	$21.99	$24.92	51	$40,000	$47,300	$52,000
Employer								
self-employed	6				2			
for-profit	29	$16.83	$20.00	$23.56	18			
nonprofit (other than government)	88	$18.62	$20.61	$24.03	47	$38,200	$42,200	$49,600
government	11				8			
Responsibilities								
director, manager or higher	10				8			
supervise 1+ employees	43	$18.58	$20.67	$25.00	27	$38,200	$40,000	$52,000
supervise none	93	$18.08	$20.67	$24.04	49	$36,500	$42,200	$48,200
have budget responsibility	17				10			
no budget responsibility	115	$18.27	$20.67	$24.04	63	$37,000	$42,000	$49,000

Note: Results not shown if fewer than 25 valid values.

Exhibit 7.5

Compensation: Clinical Dietitian, Specialist — Oncology

In addition to the duties described for the Clinical Dietitian, provides medical nutrition therapy for inpatients in a specialty area (devotes more than 50% of time to this specialty).

	HOURLY WAGE				TOTAL CASH COMPENSATION (those employed full time, 1+ years)			
	# answering	-- percentiles --			# answering	-- percentiles --		
		25th	50th	75th		25th	50th	75th
TOTAL	70	$16.96	$19.60	$22.60	55	$35,400	$40,100	$46,500
Years In Field								
20+ years	16				12			
10 - 19 years	16				12			
5 - 9 years	12				8			
< 5 years	26	$15.56	$16.83	$19.03	23			
Years In Position								
10+ years	23				18			
5 - 9 years	8				8			
< 5 years	39	$15.87	$18.00	$20.79	29	$33,700	$36,000	$41,100
Education (Highest Degree)								
doctoral degree	1				1			
master's degree	29	$16.83	$19.48	$22.60	23			
bachelor's degree	40	$17.08	$19.59	$22.36	31	$36,000	$40,000	$45,000
associate's degree								
Credentials Held								
RD	70	$16.96	$19.60	$22.60	55	$35,400	$40,100	$46,500
DTR								
state license	39	$17.69	$19.47	$22.60	31	$36,000	$40,500	$47,500
specialty certification(s)	13				9			
Employer								
self-employed								
for-profit	20				17			
nonprofit (other than government)	45	$17.35	$20.03	$22.24	33	$35,400	$40,100	$44,100
government	4				4			
Responsibilities								
director, manager or higher	5				5			
supervise 1+ employees	20				17			
supervise none	50	$16.71	$19.23	$22.35	38	$34,800	$38,400	$46,500
have budget responsibility	4				3			
no budget responsibility	65	$16.83	$19.47	$22.23	51	$35,400	$39,900	$46,400

Note: Results not shown if fewer than 25 valid values.

Exhibit 7.6

Compensation: Clinical Dietitian, Specialist — Renal

In addition to the duties described for the Clinical Dietitian, provides medical nutrition therapy for inpatients in a specialty area (devotes more than 50% of time to this specialty).

	HOURLY WAGE				TOTAL CASH COMPENSATION (those employed full time, 1+ years)			
	# answering	-- percentiles -- 25th	50th	75th	# answering	-- percentiles -- 25th	50th	75th
TOTAL	216	$19.23	$21.15	$24.00	133	$38,400	$45,000	$50,000
Years In Field								
20+ years	84	$20.19	$21.94	$24.31	55	$41,500	$47,000	$51,500
10 - 19 years	45	$20.19	$22.09	$25.00	28	$42,500	$45,500	$52,000
5 - 9 years	43	$19.00	$20.19	$22.26	20			
< 5 years	42	$16.78	$18.00	$19.90	29	$36,300	$37,800	$43,000
Years In Position								
10+ years	55	$21.03	$23.08	$26.37	41	$42,100	$46,000	$52,500
5 - 9 years	49	$19.98	$21.15	$23.08	26	$42,000	$46,400	$48,800
< 5 years	112	$17.79	$20.00	$23.33	66	$37,200	$41,000	$47,900
Education (Highest Degree)								
doctoral degree								
master's degree	86	$19.27	$21.57	$24.75	49	$39,600	$45,000	$51,000
bachelor's degree	128	$19.02	$21.03	$23.56	83	$38,000	$44,000	$49,000
associate's degree	2				1			
Credentials Held								
RD	215	$19.23	$21.15	$24.00	133	$38,400	$45,000	$50,000
DTR	1							
state license	110	$19.21	$21.07	$23.08	70	$38,000	$44,000	$48,500
specialty certification(s)	42	$20.17	$21.57	$24.52	32	$39,600	$46,000	$50,600
Employer								
self-employed	3							
for-profit	158	$19.17	$21.15	$24.00	96	$38,000	$45,000	$50,000
nonprofit (other than government)	44	$18.13	$20.73	$23.21	30	$37,400	$44,000	$48,400
government	5				5			
Responsibilities								
director, manager or higher	6				4			
supervise 1+ employees	24				19			
supervise none	192	$19.23	$21.15	$23.96	114	$38,000	$45,000	$50,000
have budget responsibility	1							
no budget responsibility	214	$19.21	$21.15	$24.01	133	$38,400	$45,000	$50,000

Note: Results not shown if fewer than 25 valid values.

Exhibit 7.7

Compensation: Clinical Dietitian, Specialist — Other

In addition to the duties described for the Clinical Dietitian, provides medical nutrition therapy for inpatients in a specialty area (devotes more than 50% of time to this specialty).

	HOURLY WAGE				TOTAL CASH COMPENSATION (those employed full time, 1+ years)			
	# answering	-- percentiles -- 25th	50th	75th	# answering	-- percentiles -- 25th	50th	75th
TOTAL	141	$18.27	$20.19	$23.08	89	$37,000	$41,000	$46,000
Years In Field								
20+ years	51	$19.71	$21.98	$25.96	30	$40,000	$44,100	$50,000
10 - 19 years	31	$19.23	$20.25	$23.39	19			
5 - 9 years	26	$16.30	$18.06	$21.83	18			
< 5 years	33	$17.01	$18.51	$20.86	22			
Years In Position								
10+ years	43	$20.00	$23.02	$25.49	28	$40,000	$44,800	$49,700
5 - 9 years	27	$19.23	$21.55	$24.67	17			
< 5 years	71	$16.83	$19.23	$20.91	44	$35,100	$39,000	$42,400
Education (Highest Degree)								
doctoral degree	2				1			
master's degree	61	$19.23	$21.00	$24.58	38	$40,000	$42,500	$47,800
bachelor's degree	77	$17.41	$19.71	$22.22	49	$35,700	$40,000	$45,000
associate's degree								
Credentials Held								
RD	137	$18.27	$20.19	$23.08	86	$37,000	$41,000	$46,300
DTR	2				2			
state license	71	$17.95	$20.05	$22.12	43	$37,000	$41,000	$45,300
specialty certification(s)	15				11			
Employer								
self-employed	3				2			
for-profit	39	$18.34	$20.67	$23.44	17			
nonprofit (other than government)	59	$18.99	$20.19	$22.12	41	$37,000	$41,000	$45,600
government	39	$16.83	$19.71	$24.04	28	$37,000	$41,700	$48,100
Responsibilities								
director, manager or higher	15				9			
supervise 1+ employees	51	$18.34	$20.19	$22.44	37	$35,900	$40,500	$44,800
supervise none	90	$17.74	$20.34	$23.17	52	$38,000	$41,200	$47,400
have budget responsibility	10				7			
no budget responsibility	129	$17.69	$20.19	$23.05	82	$36,700	$40,800	$45,500

Note: Results not shown if fewer than 25 valid values.

Exhibit 7.8

Compensation: Pediatric/Neonatal Dietitian

Performs nutrition assessments and consults for pediatric patients. Develops, implements, and monitors effectiveness of age-appropriate nutrition care plans. Provides nutrition counseling and education.

| | HOURLY WAGE | | | | TOTAL CASH COMPENSATION (those employed full time, 1+ years) | | | |
| | # answering | -- percentiles -- | | | # answering | -- percentiles -- | | |
		25th	50th	75th		25th	50th	75th
TOTAL	165	$17.50	$19.71	$22.20	108	$36,300	$41,000	$46,900
Years In Field								
20+ years	*25	$19.95	$22.28	$24.93	13			
10 - 19 years	49	$19.53	$21.15	$23.80	28	$41,100	$44,200	$48,500
5 - 9 years	35	$18.75	$19.71	$21.00	22			
< 5 years	56	$16.37	$17.64	$19.39	45	$34,000	$36,500	$39,300
Years In Position								
10+ years	39	$20.83	$22.36	$24.66	25	$43,500	$47,200	$50,000
5 - 9 years	30	$19.23	$20.19	$22.76	14			
< 5 years	96	$16.67	$18.27	$20.19	69	$34,700	$38,000	$41,300
Education (Highest Degree)								
doctoral degree	3				3			
master's degree	76	$18.75	$21.15	$23.87	45	$38,500	$43,100	$48,000
bachelor's degree	86	$16.42	$19.10	$20.49	60	$34,400	$39,000	$42,600
associate's degree								
Credentials Held								
RD	165	$17.50	$19.71	$22.20	108	$36,300	$41,000	$46,900
DTR								
state license	95	$17.00	$19.47	$21.63	67	$36,000	$39,900	$45,800
specialty certification(s)	56	$19.71	$21.63	$24.40	37	$41,500	$46,800	$50,000
Employer								
self-employed	1							
for-profit	41	$16.96	$19.45	$21.63	27	$34,700	$40,100	$46,000
nonprofit (other than government)	108	$18.27	$19.71	$22.60	70	$37,000	$40,800	$46,600
government	13				10			
Responsibilities								
director, manager or higher	9				8			
supervise 1+ employees	51	$18.75	$20.19	$24.04	34	$38,800	$41,800	$50,000
supervise none	114	$17.31	$19.40	$21.91	74	$36,000	$40,300	$45,200
have budget responsibility	4				3			
no budget responsibility	159	$17.31	$19.71	$22.12	105	$36,200	$41,000	$46,800

Note: Results not shown if fewer than 25 valid values.

Exhibit 7.9

Compensation: Nutrition Support Dietitian

Obtains and interprets nutrition assessment data to triage critically ill patients. Develops and implements individualized nutrition support care plans. Monitors nutritional status of patients receiving nutrition support.

	HOURLY WAGE				TOTAL CASH COMPENSATION (those employed full time, 1+ years)			
	# answering	-- percentiles -- 25th	50th	75th	# answering	-- percentiles -- 25th	50th	75th
TOTAL	202	$19.66	$21.79	$24.72	156	$40,000	$45,100	$52,000
Years In Field								
20+ years	47	$21.85	$24.04	$26.44	34	$45,100	$50,400	$56,000
10 - 19 years	77	$20.00	$22.25	$24.86	54	$41,400	$47,000	$52,000
5 - 9 years	49	$19.23	$20.96	$23.56	41	$40,000	$44,000	$49,700
< 5 years	29	$16.78	$18.97	$20.67	27	$35,000	$39,500	$41,600
Years In Position								
10+ years	84	$20.80	$24.04	$26.37	63	$43,000	$50,000	$56,000
5 - 9 years	47	$19.38	$21.15	$23.56	35	$40,000	$44,000	$48,000
< 5 years	69	$18.13	$20.00	$23.01	58	$36,000	$40,900	$48,500
Education (Highest Degree)								
doctoral degree								
master's degree	87	$20.51	$23.56	$25.58	64	$42,600	$48,300	$54,900
bachelor's degree	114	$19.21	$20.98	$23.17	91	$39,500	$42,600	$50,300
associate's degree	1				1			
Credentials Held								
RD	201	$19.71	$21.83	$24.72	155	$40,000	$45,200	$52,000
DTR	1				1			
state license	91	$19.98	$22.25	$24.72	71	$40,500	$46,000	$52,000
specialty certification(s)	124	$20.02	$22.04	$24.52	99	$41,000	$45,700	$51,900
Employer								
self-employed	1				1			
for-profit	55	$19.33	$21.57	$24.43	39	$39,800	$42,500	$50,000
nonprofit (other than government)	119	$19.47	$21.15	$23.56	89	$40,000	$44,000	$49,000
government	22				22			
Responsibilities								
director, manager or higher	10				6			
supervise 1+ employees	75	$19.71	$22.10	$24.52	57	$40,000	$44,900	$52,000
supervise none	125	$19.49	$21.63	$24.62	98	$40,000	$45,200	$51,900
have budget responsibility	8				7			
no budget responsibility	191	$19.51	$21.63	$24.52	147	$40,000	$45,000	$51,500

Note: Results not shown if fewer than 25 valid values.

Exhibit 7.10

Compensation: Outpatient Dietitian, General

Assesses the nutritional health of outpatients. Develops and implements individualized care plans. Provides nutrition education to individuals and groups.

	HOURLY WAGE				TOTAL CASH COMPENSATION (those employed full time, 1+ years)			
	# answering	-- percentiles -- 25th	50th	75th	# answering	-- percentiles -- 25th	50th	75th
TOTAL	332	$18.20	$20.99	$24.06	155	$37,000	$42,300	$48,900
Years In Field								
20+ years	106	$19.95	$22.06	$25.01	47	$42,000	$46,400	$53,300
10 - 19 years	86	$19.79	$22.41	$25.55	29	$40,000	$46,700	$52,700
5 - 9 years	66	$18.11	$19.42	$22.18	35	$37,800	$40,200	$45,500
< 5 years	72	$16.53	$18.04	$20.67	42	$34,300	$37,200	$42,300
Years In Position								
10+ years	105	$20.30	$22.84	$25.00	49	$42,400	$48,000	$53,200
5 - 9 years	57	$18.73	$21.84	$25.54	31	$37,400	$42,000	$48,900
< 5 years	170	$17.30	$19.41	$22.12	75	$35,000	$39,500	$44,200
Education (Highest Degree)								
doctoral degree								
master's degree	146	$19.00	$21.65	$25.42	67	$38,000	$43,300	$52,500
bachelor's degree	183	$17.31	$20.19	$23.08	86	$36,000	$41,700	$46,700
associate's degree	1				1			
Credentials Held								
RD	330	$18.21	$20.99	$24.08	153	$37,100	$42,300	$49,200
DTR	1				1			
state license	158	$17.79	$20.19	$23.08	77	$36,500	$42,000	$46,600
specialty certification(s)	68	$20.00	$22.17	$25.18	36	$41,700	$47,400	$51,300
Employer								
self-employed	18				2			
for-profit	84	$17.28	$19.32	$23.52	37	$34,700	$38,000	$47,000
nonprofit (other than government)	166	$18.27	$20.43	$23.18	75	$37,800	$42,200	$48,000
government	60	$20.19	$23.07	$25.64	37	$40,900	$45,000	$51,500
Responsibilities								
director, manager or higher	26	$18.96	$22.16	$28.27	17			
supervise 1+ employees	54	$18.15	$21.36	$25.12	33	$35,000	$44,100	$52,500
supervise none	278	$18.19	$20.94	$24.04	122	$37,400	$42,100	$48,100
have budget responsibility	27	$17.45	$20.67	$25.00	15			
no budget responsibility	302	$18.25	$21.00	$24.04	139	$37,100	$42,300	$48,300

Note: Results not shown if fewer than 25 valid values.

Exhibit 7.11

Compensation: Outpatient Dietitian, Specialist — Cardiac Rehabilitation

In addition to the duties described for the Outpatient Dietitian, provides medical nutrition therapy for outpatients in a specialty area (devotes more than 50% of time to this specialty).

	HOURLY WAGE				TOTAL CASH COMPENSATION (those employed full time, 1+ years)			
	# answering	-- percentiles -- 25th	50th	75th	# answering	-- percentiles -- 25th	50th	75th
TOTAL	39	$18.13	$19.39	$23.21	14			
Years In Field								
20+ years	14				3			
10 - 19 years	11				4			
5 - 9 years	10				5			
< 5 years	4				2			
Years In Position								
10+ years	12				3			
5 - 9 years	9				4			
< 5 years	18				7			
Education (Highest Degree)								
doctoral degree	1				1			
master's degree	24				9			
bachelor's degree	14				4			
associate's degree								
Credentials Held								
RD	39	$18.13	$19.39	$23.21	14			
DTR								
state license	22				8			
specialty certification(s)	7				3			
Employer								
self-employed	1							
for-profit	11				5			
nonprofit (other than government)	26	$18.83	$19.70	$24.47	9			
government								
Responsibilities								
director, manager or higher	1							
supervise 1+ employees	9				6			
supervise none	30	$17.95	$19.23	$23.24	8			
have budget responsibility	4				3			
no budget responsibility	34	$18.00	$19.23	$23.05	10			

Note: Results not shown if fewer than 25 valid values.

Exhibit 7.12

Compensation: Outpatient Dietitian, Specialist — Diabetes

In addition to the duties described for the Outpatient Dietitian, provides medical nutrition therapy for outpatients in a specialty area (devotes more than 50% of time to this specialty).

	HOURLY WAGE				TOTAL CASH COMPENSATION (those employed full time, 1+ years)			
	# answering	-- percentiles -- 25th	50th	75th	# answering	-- percentiles -- 25th	50th	75th
TOTAL	345	$19.23	$21.15	$24.04	171	$39,000	$44,000	$49,400
Years In Field								
20+ years	124	$20.61	$22.44	$25.00	58	$42,200	$45,600	$54,900
10 - 19 years	103	$19.74	$21.39	$24.04	48	$40,000	$46,000	$50,000
5 - 9 years	70	$18.34	$20.19	$22.18	35	$38,000	$40,500	$45,000
< 5 years	47	$16.31	$18.00	$21.63	29	$33,600	$37,100	$42,000
Years In Position								
10+ years	97	$20.60	$22.50	$25.29	49	$43,300	$46,000	$53,900
5 - 9 years	78	$19.78	$21.63	$23.72	36	$40,200	$44,300	$48,400
< 5 years	169	$17.82	$20.43	$23.09	86	$36,600	$40,500	$48,000
Education (Highest Degree)								
doctoral degree	5				1			
master's degree	140	$19.28	$21.63	$24.44	66	$40,000	$45,200	$50,000
bachelor's degree	199	$18.28	$21.00	$23.50	104	$37,600	$42,800	$48,000
associate's degree								
Credentials Held								
RD	343	$19.23	$21.15	$24.04	171	$39,000	$44,000	$49,400
DTR								
state license	176	$18.55	$20.73	$23.54	89	$38,000	$41,600	$47,500
specialty certification(s)	253	$19.78	$21.86	$24.24	128	$40,200	$44,800	$50,000
Employer								
self-employed	16				2			
for-profit	90	$19.23	$22.06	$25.00	44	$40,100	$46,000	$52,300
nonprofit (other than government)	214	$19.23	$20.98	$23.50	108	$38,100	$42,000	$46,900
government	20				15			
Responsibilities								
director, manager or higher	27	$19.23	$22.00	$26.44	15			
supervise 1+ employees	79	$19.25	$21.90	$24.04	46	$40,000	$44,800	$50,000
supervise none	265	$19.22	$21.03	$23.92	125	$38,000	$43,400	$48,800
have budget responsibility	35	$20.00	$22.00	$25.00	24			
no budget responsibility	307	$19.23	$21.15	$23.80	146	$38,000	$43,900	$49,100

Note: Results not shown if fewer than 25 valid values.

Exhibit 7.13

Compensation: Outpatient Dietitian, Specialist — Pediatrics

In addition to the duties described for the Outpatient Dietitian, provides medical nutrition therapy for outpatients in a specialty area (devotes more than 50% of time to this specialty).

| | HOURLY WAGE | | | | TOTAL CASH COMPENSATION (those employed full time, 1+ years) | | | |
	# answering	25th	50th	75th	# answering	25th	50th	75th
		-- percentiles --				-- percentiles --		
TOTAL	59	$18.99	$22.05	$24.57	36	$40,000	$43,900	$52,000
Years In Field								
20+ years	14				7			
10 - 19 years	22				13			
5 - 9 years	9				5			
< 5 years	14				11			
Years In Position								
10+ years	16				12			
5 - 9 years	15				8			
< 5 years	28	$17.79	$20.23	$22.66	16			
Education (Highest Degree)								
doctoral degree	2				2			
master's degree	30	$19.35	$22.08	$24.63	19			
bachelor's degree	26	$17.80	$21.72	$24.04	15			
associate's degree								
Credentials Held								
RD	58	$18.97	$22.05	$24.54	35	$40,000	$43,300	$52,000
DTR								
state license	33	$18.20	$21.00	$24.04	19			
specialty certification(s)	11				5			
Employer								
self-employed	2				1			
for-profit	17				9			
nonprofit (other than government)	25	$18.76	$22.44	$25.72	12			
government	14				13			
Responsibilities								
director, manager or higher	9				7			
supervise 1+ employees	15				12			
supervise none	44	$17.85	$21.17	$23.83	24			
have budget responsibility	12				9			
no budget responsibility	46	$17.95	$21.37	$23.40	26	$38,300	$42,400	$50,400

Note: Results not shown if fewer than 25 valid values.

Exhibit 7.14

Compensation: Outpatient Dietitian, Specialist — Renal

In addition to the duties described for the Outpatient Dietitian, provides medical nutrition therapy for outpatients in a specialty area (devotes more than 50% of time to this specialty).

| | HOURLY WAGE | | | | TOTAL CASH COMPENSATION (those employed full time, 1+ years) | | | |
| | # answering | -- percentiles -- | | | # answering | -- percentiles -- | | |
		25th	50th	75th		25th	50th	75th
TOTAL	245	$19.86	$22.00	$24.39	144	$41,300	$46,000	$52,000
Years In Field								
20+ years	93	$21.49	$23.08	$25.02	62	$45,700	$50,100	$55,400
10 - 19 years	72	$20.18	$21.96	$24.65	33	$41,800	$45,000	$51,400
5 - 9 years	41	$19.53	$21.03	$22.86	24			
< 5 years	38	$16.35	$18.70	$22.94	25	$34,000	$38,800	$49,200
Years In Position								
10+ years	70	$21.57	$23.29	$24.82	43	$46,000	$50,000	$53,000
5 - 9 years	57	$20.13	$21.94	$24.64	32	$41,900	$45,700	$52,000
< 5 years	118	$18.45	$21.07	$23.08	69	$37,500	$44,000	$49,300
Education (Highest Degree)								
doctoral degree								
master's degree	110	$20.00	$22.36	$24.75	66	$41,500	$47,300	$52,100
bachelor's degree	134	$19.75	$21.99	$24.04	77	$41,200	$45,700	$51,800
associate's degree								
Credentials Held								
RD	242	$19.85	$22.00	$24.23	142	$41,200	$46,000	$52,000
DTR	2				1			
state license	137	$19.31	$21.50	$23.54	87	$39,500	$45,300	$50,300
specialty certification(s)	37	$21.26	$23.29	$24.82	24			
Employer								
self-employed	8				2			
for-profit	179	$19.87	$22.00	$24.75	105	$41,300	$46,500	$52,000
nonprofit (other than government)	47	$19.23	$21.15	$22.99	31	$39,000	$44,500	$49,000
government	3				2			
Responsibilities								
director, manager or higher	16				12			
supervise 1+ employees	26	$21.63	$22.78	$24.65	22			
supervise none	219	$19.50	$21.98	$24.42	122	$39,500	$45,400	$51,800
have budget responsibility	6				5			
no budget responsibility	238	$19.85	$22.00	$24.23	138	$40,800	$45,800	$52,000

Note: Results not shown if fewer than 25 valid values.

Exhibit 7.15

Compensation: Outpatient Dietitian, Specialist — Weight Management

In addition to the duties described for the Outpatient Dietitian, provides medical nutrition therapy for outpatients in a specialty area (devotes more than 50% of time to this specialty).

	HOURLY WAGE				TOTAL CASH COMPENSATION (those employed full time, 1+ years)			
	# answering	-- percentiles -- 25th	50th	75th	# answering	-- percentiles -- 25th	50th	75th
TOTAL	55	$17.31	$19.23	$21.63	28	$36,000	$39,500	$43,800
Years In Field								
20+ years	9				6			
10 - 19 years	21				6			
5 - 9 years	13				7			
< 5 years	12				9			
Years In Position								
10+ years	12				5			
5 - 9 years	9				3			
< 5 years	34	$17.25	$18.99	$20.74	20			
Education (Highest Degree)								
doctoral degree	1							
master's degree	23				11			
bachelor's degree	30	$16.95	$19.23	$20.96	17			
associate's degree	1							
Credentials Held								
RD	51	$17.78	$19.23	$21.22	27	$36,000	$39,000	$43,300
DTR	2							
state license	30	$17.30	$18.85	$20.74	16			
specialty certification(s)	4				2			
Employer								
self-employed	6				4			
for-profit	17				8			
nonprofit (other than government)	24				13			
government	6				2			
Responsibilities								
director, manager or higher	7				2			
supervise 1+ employees	17				10			
supervise none	38	$17.91	$19.23	$21.32	18			
have budget responsibility	6				3			
no budget responsibility	49	$17.54	$19.23	$21.84	25	$35,500	$40,000	$43,700

Note: Results not shown if fewer than 25 valid values.

Exhibit 7.16

Compensation: Outpatient Dietitian, Specialist — Other

In addition to the duties described for the Outpatient Dietitian, provides medical nutrition therapy for outpatients in a specialty area (devotes more than 50% of time to this specialty).

	HOURLY WAGE				TOTAL CASH COMPENSATION (those employed full time, 1+ years)			
	# answering	-- percentiles -- 25th	50th	75th	# answering	-- percentiles -- 25th	50th	75th
TOTAL	51	$18.03	$22.00	$25.00	19			
Years In Field								
20+ years	21				6			
10 - 19 years	11				2			
5 - 9 years	8				3			
< 5 years	11				8			
Years In Position								
10+ years	16				6			
5 - 9 years	10				2			
< 5 years	25	$16.92	$19.97	$25.12	11			
Education (Highest Degree)								
doctoral degree								
master's degree	26	$17.97	$22.63	$25.68	12			
bachelor's degree	25	$18.13	$20.19	$23.30	7			
associate's degree								
Credentials Held								
RD	50	$18.21	$22.06	$25.00	18			
DTR	1				1			
state license	33	$18.15	$22.00	$24.83	13			
specialty certification(s)	7				4			
Employer								
self-employed	8				2			
for-profit	13				6			
nonprofit (other than government)	27	$17.26	$21.45	$23.80	9			
government	2				2			
Responsibilities								
director, manager or higher	9				2			
supervise 1+ employees	3				1			
supervise none	48	$18.09	$21.73	$25.00	18			
have budget responsibility	5				1			
no budget responsibility	46	$17.95	$20.61	$24.19	18			

Note: Results not shown if fewer than 25 valid values.

Exhibit 7.17

Compensation: Home Care Dietitian

Provides nutrition services to patients in a home care setting. Consults with case managers and physicians on screening and assessment of patients. Monitors and evaluates nutrition care of high-risk patients.

		HOURLY WAGE			TOTAL CASH COMPENSATION (those employed full time, 1+ years)			
	# answering	-- percentiles --			# answering	-- percentiles --		
		25th	50th	75th		25th	50th	75th
TOTAL	68	$20.00	$24.43	$27.50	20			
Years In Field								
20+ years	28	$21.40	$26.26	$28.63	8			
10 - 19 years	21				5			
5 - 9 years	7				1			
< 5 years	12				6			
Years In Position								
10+ years	16				9			
5 - 9 years	20				4			
< 5 years	32	$18.91	$21.84	$25.00	7			
Education (Highest Degree)								
doctoral degree	1							
master's degree	27	$21.00	$23.81	$26.50	7			
bachelor's degree	40	$19.23	$24.81	$28.30	13			
associate's degree								
Credentials Held								
RD	67	$20.00	$24.63	$27.69	20			
DTR	1				0			
state license	29	$19.02	$21.74	$27.85	7			
specialty certification(s)	14				4			
Employer								
self-employed	6				1			
for-profit	24				7			
nonprofit (other than government)	26	$20.40	$24.43	$28.85	4			
government	10				7			
Responsibilities								
director, manager or higher	9				3			
supervise 1+ employees	5				4			
supervise none	63	$20.00	$24.63	$27.69	16			
have budget responsibility	3							
no budget responsibility	65	$20.00	$24.63	$27.85	20			

Note: Results not shown if fewer than 25 valid values.

Exhibit 7.18

Compensation: Clinical Dietitian, Long Term Care

Develops and implements nutrition care plans for residents. Documents progress and recommendations. Provides nutrition education for residents, families, and staff. May consult with foodservice staff on food preparation, service, and delivery. May provide services as a consultant to more than one facility or be employed by single facility.

| | HOURLY WAGE | | | | TOTAL CASH COMPENSATION (those employed full time, 1+ years) | | | |
	# answering	25th	50th	75th	# answering	25th	50th	75th
		-- percentiles --				-- percentiles --		
TOTAL	1084	$18.99	$21.99	$26.92	572	$37,200	$43,000	$50,000
Years In Field								
20+ years	363	$20.67	$25.00	$31.73	168	$43,200	$50,000	$57,800
10 - 19 years	311	$19.23	$22.72	$28.02	145	$37,000	$42,000	$50,000
5 - 9 years	207	$18.99	$21.63	$25.00	119	$38,000	$43,000	$49,000
< 5 years	200	$16.41	$18.75	$21.15	139	$33,700	$38,000	$42,000
Years In Position								
10+ years	348	$20.19	$24.07	$31.83	168	$41,100	$48,500	$56,000
5 - 9 years	221	$19.28	$23.08	$27.44	116	$38,400	$44,300	$51,900
< 5 years	513	$18.01	$20.19	$24.47	288	$36,000	$40,100	$45,400
Education (Highest Degree)								
doctoral degree	7				4			
master's degree	353	$20.00	$24.04	$30.00	178	$39,500	$45,000	$53,300
bachelor's degree	681	$18.75	$21.50	$25.98	358	$37,500	$42,400	$49,900
associate's degree	40	$13.94	$15.32	$18.13	31	$27,600	$31,300	$37,000
Credentials Held								
RD	1018	$19.23	$22.61	$27.59	518	$38,200	$43,300	$50,600
DTR	56	$14.18	$15.39	$18.49	45	$28,900	$32,000	$38,000
state license	574	$19.23	$22.65	$28.85	281	$38,000	$43,500	$50,100
specialty certification(s)	49	$19.23	$24.04	$29.74	22			
Employer								
self-employed	286	$23.08	$29.89	$35.78	55	$45,000	$52,500	$75,000
for-profit	452	$18.75	$21.00	$24.12	286	$37,900	$42,600	$50,000
nonprofit (other than government)	220	$17.20	$20.00	$23.56	132	$34,600	$40,000	$45,300
government	113	$17.86	$21.31	$24.01	95	$37,500	$43,800	$50,000
Responsibilities								
director, manager or higher	321	$19.23	$22.66	$27.83	206	$39,000	$44,900	$52,000
supervise 1+ employees	624	$19.00	$21.63	$26.44	360	$37,900	$43,000	$50,000
supervise none	454	$18.62	$22.78	$27.69	210	$36,300	$43,000	$50,000
have budget responsibility	154	$18.99	$21.63	$26.51	111	$38,600	$43,300	$52,000
no budget responsibility	886	$18.98	$22.00	$27.00	443	$36,700	$43,000	$50,000

Note: Results not shown if fewer than 25 valid values.

Exhibit 7.19

Compensation: Dietetic Technician, Long Term Care

Performs nutrition screening and routine assessments, and provides basic nutrition care. Monitors resident satisfaction and tolerance of meals. May monitor food production and meal service.

	HOURLY WAGE				TOTAL CASH COMPENSATION (those employed full time, 1+ years)			
	# answering	-- percentiles -- 25th	50th	75th	# answering	-- percentiles -- 25th	50th	75th
TOTAL	232	$12.50	$14.25	$15.91	147	$26,000	$29,000	$33,000
Years In Field								
20+ years	43	$13.22	$14.71	$17.07	33	$27,700	$30,600	$35,900
10 - 19 years	68	$12.98	$14.42	$16.31	39	$28,000	$30,000	$35,000
5 - 9 years	75	$12.12	$13.46	$15.38	49	$25,000	$28,000	$32,000
< 5 years	46	$11.70	$13.51	$15.43	26	$23,800	$27,200	$31,600
Years In Position								
10+ years	55	$13.47	$14.42	$16.67	43	$28,000	$30,000	$35,000
5 - 9 years	63	$12.31	$14.31	$16.35	39	$25,000	$28,500	$32,800
< 5 years	114	$12.04	$13.85	$15.87	65	$25,500	$28,100	$32,600
Education (Highest Degree)								
doctoral degree								
master's degree	4				3			
bachelor's degree	50	$12.82	$14.42	$16.82	26	$26,800	$29,300	$36,300
associate's degree	178	$12.10	$14.00	$15.68	118	$26,000	$29,000	$32,000
Credentials Held								
RD	2				2			
DTR	229	$12.50	$14.24	$15.89	144	$26,000	$29,000	$32,600
state license	11				6			
specialty certification(s)	11				9			
Employer								
self-employed	4				2			
for-profit	97	$12.35	$14.30	$16.71	61	$25,500	$29,700	$33,600
nonprofit (other than government)	110	$12.44	$14.10	$15.38	67	$26,000	$28,900	$32,000
government	18				16			
Responsibilities								
director, manager or higher	49	$13.43	$15.38	$17.51	38	$29,700	$32,400	$37,100
supervise 1+ employees	135	$12.98	$14.42	$16.68	94	$27,000	$31,000	$35,100
supervise none	95	$12.00	$13.50	$15.00	52	$24,000	$27,200	$29,800
have budget responsibility	47	$12.50	$14.90	$17.31	38	$28,000	$32,100	$37,100
no budget responsibility	174	$12.47	$13.97	$15.63	104	$25,200	$28,200	$31,300

Note: Results not shown if fewer than 25 valid values.

Exhibit 7.20

Compensation: WIC Nutritionist

Contributes to the development, implementation, and evaluation of the nutrition education component of the WIC program. Provides nutrition therapy and education for WIC clients. Offers technical assistance to WIC staff. May provide supervision and training for WIC staff.

	HOURLY WAGE				TOTAL CASH COMPENSATION (those employed full time, 1+ years)			
	# answering	-- percentiles -- 25th	50th	75th	# answering	-- percentiles -- 25th	50th	75th
TOTAL	585	$15.14	$17.79	$21.59	380	$32,000	$37,400	$45,700
Years In Field								
20+ years	155	$17.31	$20.82	$24.48	100	$38,600	$45,500	$51,400
10 - 19 years	172	$15.64	$18.73	$22.38	112	$32,600	$38,100	$45,200
5 - 9 years	133	$14.66	$16.83	$20.00	86	$30,700	$35,000	$40,300
< 5 years	124	$13.46	$15.77	$17.39	81	$28,500	$32,600	$37,500
Years In Position								
10+ years	177	$16.20	$19.75	$24.01	118	$35,000	$42,100	$50,000
5 - 9 years	167	$15.00	$18.19	$21.42	105	$31,000	$37,000	$45,000
< 5 years	241	$14.42	$16.59	$20.19	157	$30,300	$34,900	$42,300
Education (Highest Degree)								
doctoral degree	1							
master's degree	190	$16.81	$19.87	$24.15	121	$35,100	$43,000	$51,500
bachelor's degree	326	$15.17	$17.66	$21.37	220	$31,400	$36,300	$44,900
associate's degree	65	$12.02	$13.41	$15.50	37	$24,500	$28,400	$32,800
Credentials Held								
RD	478	$16.16	$19.15	$22.18	313	$33,400	$40,000	$47,000
DTR	97	$12.02	$13.53	$15.63	59	$25,000	$28,100	$32,500
state license	250	$15.51	$17.23	$21.00	159	$32,000	$36,400	$44,500
specialty certification(s)	32	$17.79	$21.09	$25.65	21			
Employer								
self-employed	5							
for-profit	8				5			
nonprofit (other than government)	174	$14.42	$17.99	$21.53	111	$31,100	$36,800	$45,000
government	382	$15.38	$17.79	$21.63	258	$32,000	$38,000	$45,900
Responsibilities								
director, manager or higher	53	$16.91	$20.23	$25.58	45	$35,000	$43,800	$51,300
supervise 1+ employees	343	$16.59	$19.71	$23.25	247	$34,900	$41,000	$49,000
supervise none	240	$13.48	$15.82	$18.46	132	$28,000	$32,000	$36,200
have budget responsibility	108	$17.00	$20.10	$24.02	75	$35,100	$41,600	$50,000
no budget responsibility	456	$14.91	$17.06	$20.97	288	$31,100	$36,000	$43,900

Note: Results not shown if fewer than 25 valid values.

Exhibit 7.21

Compensation: Public Health Nutritionist

Contributes to the planning, development, coordination, and evaluation of public health nutrition programs. Assesses community nutritional needs and develops related standards and services. May counsel patients on normal and therapeutic nutrition. May provide supervision and training for public health department staff.

| | HOURLY WAGE | | | | TOTAL CASH COMPENSATION (those employed full time, 1+ years) | | | |
	# answering	-- percentiles -- 25th	50th	75th	# answering	-- percentiles -- 25th	50th	75th
TOTAL	317	$18.44	$22.60	$27.32	224	$38,000	$45,800	$56,000
Years In Field								
20+ years	131	$21.03	$24.52	$29.38	97	$44,800	$52,000	$62,000
10 - 19 years	90	$19.95	$22.43	$26.28	62	$39,800	$44,400	$57,400
5 - 9 years	43	$17.31	$21.11	$26.44	28	$35,000	$40,800	$50,700
< 5 years	53	$15.88	$17.79	$20.40	37	$32,600	$36,500	$44,500
Years In Position								
10+ years	116	$20.96	$23.98	$28.85	89	$42,800	$49,300	$60,000
5 - 9 years	58	$18.71	$23.44	$28.99	40	$38,400	$45,000	$57,000
< 5 years	142	$17.31	$20.65	$25.00	95	$35,000	$42,200	$52,900
Education (Highest Degree)								
doctoral degree	2				1			
master's degree	204	$20.05	$23.08	$28.85	147	$41,200	$48,000	$60,000
bachelor's degree	107	$17.13	$21.06	$25.00	74	$33,600	$42,300	$52,400
associate's degree	4				2			
Credentials Held								
RD	306	$19.14	$22.84	$27.46	218	$38,200	$46,400	$57,000
DTR	8				3			
state license	165	$18.11	$21.65	$25.30	123	$38,000	$45,200	$55,000
specialty certification(s)	39	$20.51	$22.00	$28.57	26	$43,000	$50,300	$60,300
Employer								
self-employed	7							
for-profit	8				6			
nonprofit (other than government)	53	$17.07	$20.00	$23.89	37	$35,300	$42,200	$54,200
government	249	$19.30	$23.08	$27.90	181	$40,400	$47,500	$57,700
Responsibilities								
director, manager or higher	68	$21.69	$26.08	$33.19	52	$46,000	$56,000	$70,200
supervise 1+ employees	166	$19.93	$23.56	$28.44	133	$41,100	$49,300	$60,000
supervise none	149	$17.31	$21.19	$25.44	90	$35,100	$43,000	$50,200
have budget responsibility	131	$19.22	$23.56	$28.85	101	$40,900	$49,000	$60,500
no budget responsibility	177	$17.65	$21.65	$26.02	115	$36,000	$43,600	$54,500

Note: Results not shown if fewer than 25 valid values.

Exhibit 7.22

Compensation: Cooperative Extension Educator/Specialist

Develops, implements, and evaluates educational programs and materials addressing family and community needs. Conducts family and consumer educational programs. Responds to general, family, consumer, food safety, food, and nutrition questions. May involve a faculty appointment to an affiliated university.

	HOURLY WAGE				TOTAL CASH COMPENSATION (those employed full time, 1+ years)			
	# answering	-- percentiles -- 25th	50th	75th	# answering	-- percentiles -- 25th	50th	75th
TOTAL	87	$15.00	$19.23	$24.04	52	$36,600	$45,500	$52,000
Years In Field								
20+ years	24				14			
10 - 19 years	30	$18.36	$21.88	$25.55	20			
5 - 9 years	14				5			
< 5 years	19				13			
Years In Position								
10+ years	18				14			
5 - 9 years	22				12			
< 5 years	47	$13.48	$17.79	$22.26	26	$31,300	$39,900	$49,000
Education (Highest Degree)								
doctoral degree	11				9			
master's degree	42	$17.95	$21.01	$25.00	30	$39,000	$47,500	$52,100
bachelor's degree	18				8			
associate's degree	16				5			
Credentials Held								
RD	69	$17.79	$21.63	$25.25	46	$39,800	$48,200	$53,100
DTR	17				6			
state license	27	$15.50	$22.12	$25.24	18			
specialty certification(s)	7				4			
Employer								
self-employed								
for-profit	2				1			
nonprofit (other than government)	37	$14.39	$18.12	$24.52	22			
government	44	$15.66	$21.01	$24.76	28	$39,500	$48,400	$54,400
Responsibilities								
director, manager or higher	10				8			
supervise 1+ employees	40	$18.87	$22.19	$25.54	30	$42,400	$49,100	$58,100
supervise none	47	$12.82	$16.38	$21.63	22			
have budget responsibility	44	$15.76	$19.64	$24.76	28	$38,700	$47,900	$51,500
no budget responsibility	43	$13.50	$19.23	$24.04	24			

Note: Results not shown if fewer than 25 valid values.

Exhibit 7.23

Compensation: School/Child Care Nutritionist

Plans, develops, and implements school and childcare nutrition programs and resources. Monitors and evaluates menus and foodservice programs. Consults with parents and school leaders on nutritional needs of high-risk children.

	HOURLY WAGE				TOTAL CASH COMPENSATION (those employed full time, 1+ years)			
	# answering	-- percentiles --			# answering	-- percentiles --		
		25th	50th	75th		25th	50th	75th
TOTAL	71	$18.27	$26.44	$31.89	48	$38,500	$52,900	$62,600
Years In Field								
20+ years	33	$23.56	$29.81	$32.88	27	$45,000	$60,000	$65,000
10 - 19 years	22				11			
5 - 9 years	7				4			
< 5 years	9				6			
Years In Position								
10+ years	25	$24.33	$30.48	$33.07	18			
5 - 9 years	14				12			
< 5 years	32	$15.87	$20.00	$27.64	18			
Education (Highest Degree)								
doctoral degree	1				1			
master's degree	28	$27.28	$31.57	$32.92	21			
bachelor's degree	37	$16.02	$20.57	$28.30	23			
associate's degree	5				3			
Credentials Held								
RD	60	$20.79	$28.13	$32.09	42	$45,000	$57,500	$63,800
DTR	10				6			
state license	27	$18.27	$26.44	$30.77	21			
specialty certification(s)	3				2			
Employer								
self-employed	3				1			
for-profit	4				3			
nonprofit (other than government)	23				16			
government	40	$21.63	$28.13	$32.09	28	$50,000	$58,500	$66,200
Responsibilities								
director, manager or higher	16				13			
supervise 1+ employees	39	$18.27	$28.40	$32.21	25	$38,400	$55,000	$66,800
supervise none	31	$17.70	$23.08	$29.81	22			
have budget responsibility	29	$19.24	$21.81	$31.34	22			
no budget responsibility	40	$17.72	$25.77	$31.73	25	$41,600	$57,000	$62,500

Note: Results not shown if fewer than 25 valid values.

Exhibit 7.24

Compensation: Corrections Dietitian

Plans, directs, and coordinates food and nutrition services for inmates. Monitors and evaluates menus for normal and therapeutic diets. Provides diet instructions for inmates. May supervise and train foodservice personnel.

	HOURLY WAGE				TOTAL CASH COMPENSATION (those employed full time, 1+ years)			
	# answering	-- percentiles --			# answering	-- percentiles --		
		25th	50th	75th		25th	50th	75th
TOTAL	16				12			
Years In Field								
20+ years	4				1			
10 - 19 years	6				5			
5 - 9 years	4				4			
< 5 years	2				2			
Years In Position								
10+ years	3				2			
5 - 9 years	6				4			
< 5 years	7				6			
Education (Highest Degree)								
doctoral degree								
master's degree	6				5			
bachelor's degree	10				7			
associate's degree								
Credentials Held								
RD	15				11			
DTR								
state license	11				9			
specialty certification(s)								
Employer								
self-employed								
for-profit	2				1			
nonprofit (other than government)								
government	14				11			
Responsibilities								
director, manager or higher	5				5			
supervise 1+ employees	10				8			
supervise none	6				4			
have budget responsibility	6				4			
no budget responsibility	10				8			

Note: Results not shown if fewer than 25 valid values.

Exhibit 7.25

Compensation: Nutrition Coordinator for Head Start Program

Designs and implements nutrition programs that meet the nutritional needs and feeding requirements of each child. Provides counseling to parents of children at nutritional risk. Plans menus and special meals. May supervise foodservice operations.

	# answering	HOURLY WAGE			# answering	TOTAL CASH COMPENSATION (those employed full time, 1+ years)		
		25th	50th	75th		25th	50th	75th
TOTAL	36	$13.98	$18.09	$22.11	17			
Years In Field								
20+ years	8				4			
10 - 19 years	10				5			
5 - 9 years	7				3			
< 5 years	11				5			
Years In Position								
10+ years	4				2			
5 - 9 years	9				7			
< 5 years	23				8			
Education (Highest Degree)								
doctoral degree	1							
master's degree	8				4			
bachelor's degree	24				12			
associate's degree	3				1			
Credentials Held								
RD	30	$14.92	$18.45	$23.31	14			
DTR	5				2			
state license	16				9			
specialty certification(s)	3							
Employer								
self-employed	3							
for-profit								
nonprofit (other than government)	22				11			
government	11				6			
Responsibilities								
director, manager or higher	8				4			
supervise 1+ employees	26	$14.70	$18.91	$24.01	15			
supervise none	10				2			
have budget responsibility	19				12			
no budget responsibility	17				5			

Note: Results not shown if fewer than 25 valid values.

Exhibit 7.26

Compensation: Nutritionist for Food Bank or Assistance Program

Performs client nutrition assessments and follow-ups, and refers and advocates for clients to other service providers. Conducts nutrition education workshops for clients, staff, and community groups. Monitors and evaluates nutritional content and quality assurance of food products. May supervise and train staff.

| | HOURLY WAGE | | | | TOTAL CASH COMPENSATION (those employed full time, 1+ years) | | | |
	# answering	25th	50th	75th	# answering	25th	50th	75th
		-- percentiles --				-- percentiles --		
TOTAL	26	$15.38	$17.00	$21.46	20			
Years In Field								
20+ years	7				6			
10 - 19 years	5				4			
5 - 9 years	6				4			
< 5 years	8				6			
Years In Position								
10+ years	3				3			
5 - 9 years	5				4			
< 5 years	18				13			
Education (Highest Degree)								
doctoral degree								
master's degree	16				12			
bachelor's degree	9				7			
associate's degree	1				1			
Credentials Held								
RD	23				17			
DTR	2				2			
state license	11				7			
specialty certification(s)	1				1			
Employer								
self-employed	1							
for-profit								
nonprofit (other than government)	21				16			
government	4				4			
Responsibilities								
director, manager or higher	5				4			
supervise 1+ employees	15				14			
supervise none	11				6			
have budget responsibility	14				11			
no budget responsibility	12				9			

Note: Results not shown if fewer than 25 valid values.

Exhibit 7.27

Compensation: Executive-level Professional

Plans, controls, and directs services/operations for multiple departments, product lines, or facilities. Accountable for quality of services, financial results, and achievement of organizational objectives.

| | HOURLY WAGE | | | | TOTAL CASH COMPENSATION (those employed full time, 1+ years) | | | |
| | # answering | -- percentiles -- | | | # answering | -- percentiles -- | | |
		25th	50th	75th		25th	50th	75th
TOTAL	193	$28.85	$34.86	$41.80	173	$62,400	$77,000	$90,000
Years In Field								
20+ years	121	$31.13	$36.06	$43.27	111	$69,000	$81,000	$93,000
10 - 19 years	55	$26.44	$32.21	$38.22	47	$56,000	$71,500	$92,000
5 - 9 years	14				13			
< 5 years	3				2			
Years In Position								
10+ years	95	$30.77	$38.72	$44.23	86	$65,900	$82,800	$97,100
5 - 9 years	26	$28.85	$33.89	$36.71	24			
< 5 years	72	$25.00	$31.25	$36.06	63	$55,000	$72,100	$83,000
Education (Highest Degree)								
doctoral degree	3				2			
master's degree	108	$30.77	$36.06	$43.27	99	$68,000	$79,400	$94,000
bachelor's degree	75	$26.92	$31.73	$39.90	65	$57,100	$70,000	$87,500
associate's degree	7				7			
Credentials Held								
RD	178	$29.71	$35.45	$42.37	158	$65,000	$77,600	$92,000
DTR	11				11			
state license	98	$27.28	$34.06	$40.84	86	$60,000	$75,300	$90,100
specialty certification(s)	20				18			
Employer								
self-employed	9				4			
for-profit	74	$28.63	$32.57	$36.36	68	$63,600	$74,300	$88,500
nonprofit (other than government)	66	$31.66	$36.30	$43.87	59	$68,000	$82,600	$101,000
government	43	$27.14	$35.23	$40.34	41	$55,700	$74,000	$85,200
Responsibilities								
director, manager or higher	185	$29.25	$35.10	$42.29	165	$65,000	$77,500	$90,200
supervise 1+ employees	180	$29.35	$35.16	$41.81	166	$65,000	$77,500	$90,100
supervise none	13				7			
have budget responsibility	176	$29.35	$35.28	$42.32	161	$65,000	$77,500	$91,200
no budget responsibility	16				11			

Note: Results not shown if fewer than 25 valid values.

Exhibit 7.28

Compensation: Director of Food and Nutrition Services

Plans, coordinates, and evaluates the personnel and activities of the food and nutrition services department. Directs food and equipment purchasing. Manages budget and human resource needs of staff. Develops and implements department policies and procedures.

	HOURLY WAGE				TOTAL CASH COMPENSATION (those employed full time, 1+ years)			
	# answering	-- percentiles -- 25th	50th	75th	# answering	-- percentiles -- 25th	50th	75th
TOTAL	579	$20.19	$25.07	$30.55	508	$43,000	$53,000	$64,900
Years In Field								
20+ years	311	$22.60	$27.40	$32.19	276	$48,300	$58,600	$68,500
10 - 19 years	150	$20.63	$25.00	$29.92	129	$44,100	$52,000	$64,800
5 - 9 years	78	$17.14	$20.93	$27.03	71	$36,000	$45,300	$57,000
< 5 years	39	$14.42	$17.55	$20.62	31	$32,000	$38,000	$43,700
Years In Position								
10+ years	255	$22.12	$26.92	$31.63	225	$46,700	$56,000	$67,700
5 - 9 years	113	$18.99	$24.04	$29.27	101	$40,000	$50,300	$63,100
< 5 years	209	$19.23	$24.04	$28.85	182	$42,000	$51,600	$61,700
Education (Highest Degree)								
doctoral degree	3				2			
master's degree	240	$23.18	$28.85	$33.29	211	$48,000	$60,000	$71,000
bachelor's degree	267	$20.63	$25.00	$28.85	235	$44,000	$52,200	$61,800
associate's degree	69	$14.95	$17.31	$20.40	60	$32,000	$37,100	$43,000
Credentials Held								
RD	478	$22.09	$26.44	$31.25	419	$47,000	$56,000	$66,600
DTR	92	$15.38	$18.03	$21.60	82	$32,100	$40,000	$47,300
state license	284	$20.71	$25.96	$30.77	255	$46,000	$54,900	$65,500
specialty certification(s)	58	$20.85	$25.24	$32.74	52	$45,000	$53,300	$69,800
Employer								
self-employed	6				4			
for-profit	149	$19.23	$23.56	$28.61	131	$41,000	$50,000	$63,200
nonprofit (other than government)	293	$20.65	$25.05	$30.24	261	$43,300	$53,000	$62,900
government	127	$21.63	$27.88	$33.48	108	$45,500	$59,300	$70,500
Responsibilities								
director, manager or higher	559	$20.43	$25.13	$30.77	491	$43,300	$53,500	$65,000
supervise 1+ employees	576	$20.22	$25.10	$30.56	505	$43,000	$53,000	$65,000
supervise none	1				1			
have budget responsibility	559	$20.43	$25.24	$30.77	490	$43,000	$53,500	$65,000
no budget responsibility	8				7			

Note: Results not shown if fewer than 25 valid values.

Exhibit 7.29

Compensation: Clinical Nutrition Manager

Plans, organizes, and manages clinical nutrition services. Recruits, trains, supervises, and evaluates clinical nutrition staff. Develops and implements policies and procedures. Manages human resources and budget. May also perform duties of a patient services manager.

	HOURLY WAGE				TOTAL CASH COMPENSATION (those employed full time, 1+ years)			
	# answering	-- percentiles -- 25th	50th	75th	# answering	-- percentiles -- 25th	50th	75th
TOTAL	336	$21.67	$25.00	$28.08	298	$45,000	$51,900	$59,000
Years In Field								
20+ years	146	$24.04	$26.24	$29.81	134	$49,700	$55,000	$62,600
10 - 19 years	96	$22.13	$25.00	$27.86	79	$45,600	$51,600	$58,000
5 - 9 years	62	$20.88	$24.13	$26.12	57	$43,200	$50,300	$54,000
< 5 years	32	$18.03	$19.23	$21.16	28	$37,700	$41,000	$42,000
Years In Position								
10+ years	105	$23.95	$26.25	$30.18	96	$49,000	$55,000	$64,400
5 - 9 years	67	$22.05	$24.52	$28.59	58	$45,500	$52,000	$60,100
< 5 years	162	$20.77	$24.04	$26.43	144	$43,200	$50,000	$54,100
Education (Highest Degree)								
doctoral degree	1				1			
master's degree	160	$23.32	$25.68	$28.44	140	$48,000	$52,000	$60,000
bachelor's degree	172	$20.88	$24.04	$27.01	155	$43,300	$50,000	$55,000
associate's degree	2				1			
Credentials Held								
RD	332	$21.88	$25.00	$28.14	295	$45,300	$52,000	$59,000
DTR	3				2			
state license	201	$21.53	$25.00	$27.69	182	$45,000	$51,800	$59,000
specialty certification(s)	67	$23.51	$26.25	$29.03	59	$48,800	$54,000	$60,000
Employer								
self-employed	1							
for-profit	131	$20.67	$23.53	$25.96	116	$43,000	$48,700	$54,400
nonprofit (other than government)	175	$23.08	$25.48	$28.85	155	$48,000	$52,900	$59,200
government	27	$19.87	$28.83	$31.30	26	$42,100	$60,000	$66,000
Responsibilities								
director, manager or higher	256	$21.80	$25.00	$28.08	230	$45,300	$52,000	$59,000
supervise 1+ employees	333	$21.71	$25.00	$28.12	295	$45,000	$51,900	$59,000
supervise none	2				2			
have budget responsibility	163	$22.60	$25.72	$29.13	145	$47,700	$53,000	$61,300
no budget responsibility	149	$20.81	$23.74	$26.34	131	$43,000	$49,400	$54,600

Note: Results not shown if fewer than 25 valid values.

Exhibit 7.30

Compensation: Assistant Foodservice Director

Manages daily operations of foodservice department. Directs and supervises the preparation and service of food. Recruits, trains, supervises, and evaluates foodservice staff. Assists in managing budget.

	HOURLY WAGE				TOTAL CASH COMPENSATION (those employed full time, 1+ years)			
	# answering	-- percentiles -- 25th	50th	75th	# answering	-- percentiles -- 25th	50th	75th
TOTAL	131	$18.27	$21.63	$25.96	106	$39,900	$47,000	$54,600
Years In Field								
20+ years	44	$21.56	$24.76	$30.78	39	$45,500	$53,000	$62,100
10 - 19 years	45	$18.65	$21.63	$25.48	35	$40,600	$49,800	$55,000
5 - 9 years	25	$16.43	$19.23	$23.04	18			
< 5 years	17				14			
Years In Position								
10+ years	42	$20.02	$24.24	$28.65	38	$42,900	$51,100	$59,600
5 - 9 years	26	$18.80	$23.34	$25.55	17			
< 5 years	61	$16.83	$19.50	$23.08	51	$35,500	$43,700	$53,000
Education (Highest Degree)								
doctoral degree								
master's degree	51	$19.35	$24.04	$30.77	41	$42,900	$53,500	$61,800
bachelor's degree	66	$18.38	$21.15	$24.14	53	$39,000	$45,000	$52,800
associate's degree	14				12			
Credentials Held								
RD	104	$19.08	$22.80	$26.97	84	$41,500	$49,900	$55,000
DTR	23				19			
state license	55	$18.50	$22.12	$26.20	49	$40,800	$47,000	$54,500
specialty certification(s)	7				7			
Employer								
self-employed								
for-profit	37	$16.83	$19.58	$25.02	31	$35,500	$45,000	$53,000
nonprofit (other than government)	65	$19.13	$22.36	$25.00	51	$42,000	$49,800	$58,000
government	27	$19.00	$23.56	$28.85	23			
Responsibilities								
director, manager or higher	86	$18.49	$22.43	$26.44	72	$40,700	$48,100	$55,000
supervise 1+ employees	130	$18.27	$21.54	$25.60	106	$39,900	$47,000	$54,600
supervise none								
have budget responsibility	86	$19.23	$22.55	$26.26	75	$40,800	$49,000	$55,000
no budget responsibility	33	$16.83	$20.19	$24.72	24			

Note: Results not shown if fewer than 25 valid values.

Exhibit 7.31

Compensation: School Foodservice Director

Develops, implements, and maintains the foodservice program in a school setting. Directs and monitors food procurement and storage, and food production, assembly, and service to students. Plans menus to meet required nutritional standards and student acceptance.

| | HOURLY WAGE | | | | TOTAL CASH COMPENSATION (those employed full time, 1+ years) | | | |
	# answering	25th	50th	75th	# answering	25th	50th	75th
		-- percentiles --				-- percentiles --		
TOTAL	116	$20.20	$24.83	$30.40	55	$44,000	$54,700	$70,000
Years In Field								
20+ years	53	$22.62	$26.44	$32.77	29	$50,200	$60,000	$74,000
10 - 19 years	41	$20.19	$24.09	$30.84	19			
5 - 9 years	17				5			
< 5 years	5				2			
Years In Position								
10+ years	46	$23.01	$26.68	$36.06	26	$50,100	$62,000	$75,600
5 - 9 years	25	$19.95	$25.96	$30.73	11			
< 5 years	45	$18.87	$23.44	$26.78	18			
Education (Highest Degree)								
doctoral degree								
master's degree	42	$23.11	$26.78	$32.00	19			
bachelor's degree	56	$20.74	$25.00	$31.56	28	$45,000	$57,100	$72,300
associate's degree	17				7			
Credentials Held								
RD	92	$21.61	$25.84	$32.09	45	$49,000	$58,200	$72,800
DTR	23				10			
state license	48	$20.39	$24.46	$31.20	18			
specialty certification(s)	10				6			
Employer								
self-employed								
for-profit	13				10			
nonprofit (other than government)	58	$19.90	$24.46	$30.35	17			
government	44	$20.48	$25.60	$35.01	27	$44,000	$56,000	$75,000
Responsibilities								
director, manager or higher	86	$20.65	$25.12	$30.63	43	$48,000	$57,700	$73,000
supervise 1+ employees	113	$20.20	$24.65	$30.37	52	$45,000	$54,600	$69,300
supervise none	3				3			
have budget responsibility	95	$20.65	$24.65	$30.29	47	$47,800	$56,000	$72,300
no budget responsibility	13				5			

Note: Results not shown if fewer than 25 valid values.

Exhibit 7.32

Compensation: Dietetic Technician, Foodservice Management

Oversees meal production, service, and delivery. Manages employee orientation, training, performance evaluations, scheduling, and assignment of tasks. Assures compliance with standards, policies, and procedures.

	HOURLY WAGE				TOTAL CASH COMPENSATION (those employed full time, 1+ years)			
	# answering	-- percentiles -- 25th	50th	75th	# answering	-- percentiles -- 25th	50th	75th
TOTAL	155	$13.46	$15.38	$18.43	108	$30,000	$34,000	$40,500
Years In Field								
20+ years	43	$14.42	$16.83	$19.38	35	$31,200	$35,400	$42,200
10 - 19 years	55	$14.42	$16.35	$19.69	33	$30,000	$35,000	$43,500
5 - 9 years	31	$12.02	$14.74	$17.63	21			
< 5 years	26	$13.09	$14.42	$16.48	19			
Years In Position								
10+ years	42	$14.98	$17.15	$20.67	33	$32,000	$38,000	$44,400
5 - 9 years	32	$13.04	$15.00	$18.20	25	$27,500	$30,400	$37,200
< 5 years	81	$12.98	$15.00	$18.01	50	$29,600	$32,000	$37,700
Education (Highest Degree)								
doctoral degree								
master's degree	5				5			
bachelor's degree	35	$14.42	$15.75	$19.74	27	$31,400	$36,400	$43,000
associate's degree	115	$13.23	$15.30	$18.17	76	$29,300	$32,100	$38,000
Credentials Held								
RD	14				12			
DTR	139	$13.30	$15.38	$18.27	94	$30,000	$32,900	$38,800
state license	12				11			
specialty certification(s)	16				11			
Employer								
self-employed	2							
for-profit	43	$13.46	$15.09	$18.27	37	$30,000	$32,000	$39,300
nonprofit (other than government)	79	$13.46	$15.38	$18.27	50	$30,000	$33,500	$41,200
government	29	$14.42	$17.31	$20.55	20			
Responsibilities								
director, manager or higher	58	$13.36	$15.49	$18.87	44	$30,000	$32,400	$40,500
supervise 1+ employees	143	$13.46	$15.38	$18.27	104	$30,000	$32,900	$40,500
supervise none	10				3			
have budget responsibility	67	$13.46	$15.09	$18.17	46	$30,000	$32,500	$40,700
no budget responsibility	70	$13.81	$16.74	$20.31	49	$31,000	$35,000	$42,500

Note: Results not shown if fewer than 25 valid values.

Exhibit 7.33

Compensation: Private Practice Dietitian— Patient/Client Nutrition Care

Provides medical nutrition therapy or wellness, fitness, or sports nutrition counseling for individuals or groups in a private practice setting or healthcare provider's office.

	HOURLY WAGE				TOTAL CASH COMPENSATION (those employed full time, 1+ years)			
	# answering	-- percentiles --			# answering	-- percentiles --		
		25th	50th	75th		25th	50th	75th
TOTAL	258	$16.90	$24.04	$34.34	56	$32,000	$43,000	$56,000
Years In Field								
20+ years	89	$15.50	$25.00	$32.93	15			
10 - 19 years	95	$19.83	$25.93	$37.27	16			
5 - 9 years	41	$17.15	$21.63	$26.96	10			
< 5 years	33	$14.21	$18.00	$30.63	15			
Years In Position								
10+ years	80	$20.41	$28.31	$39.77	16			
5 - 9 years	60	$15.44	$24.92	$33.32	15			
< 5 years	118	$15.97	$20.00	$28.70	25	$31,000	$40,500	$48,800
Education (Highest Degree)								
doctoral degree	8				3			
master's degree	138	$17.73	$25.00	$37.67	32	$40,100	$49,300	$67,900
bachelor's degree	106	$17.35	$23.43	$30.94	19			
associate's degree	5				1			
Credentials Held								
RD	248	$17.10	$24.53	$34.84	53	$33,500	$43,100	$56,300
DTR	8				2			
state license	122	$16.50	$23.75	$32.74	27	$31,000	$40,500	$56,000
specialty certification(s)	58	$17.49	$24.53	$32.70	19			
Employer								
self-employed	192	$17.32	$25.64	$38.39	36	$31,300	$48,100	$65,000
for-profit	48	$15.50	$20.20	$25.00	15			
nonprofit (other than government)	12				3			
government								
Responsibilities								
director, manager or higher	178	$16.79	$25.00	$37.67	36	$31,300	$46,500	$65,000
supervise 1+ employees	48	$17.36	$23.40	$30.94	22			
supervise none	210	$16.79	$24.53	$35.88	34	$32,000	$45,000	$58,800
have budget responsibility	72	$15.17	$21.93	$28.73	19			
no budget responsibility	183	$17.31	$25.00	$37.27	34	$34,300	$41,500	$52,500

Note: Results not shown if fewer than 25 valid values.

Exhibit 7.34

Compensation: Consultant — Community and/or Corporate Programs

Provides food and nutrition consultation services for community-based programs, such as meal programs, day care centers, or group homes. Develops and implements wellness events and programs for communities and/or corporations.

| | HOURLY WAGE | | | | TOTAL CASH COMPENSATION (those employed full time, 1+ years) | | | |
| | # answering | -- percentiles -- | | | # answering | -- percentiles -- | | |
		25th	50th	75th		25th	50th	75th
TOTAL	153	$19.11	$25.00	$33.15	54	$39,600	$47,100	$57,500
Years In Field								
20+ years	56	$19.25	$26.69	$33.24	18			
10 - 19 years	48	$21.17	$26.98	$38.46	17			
5 - 9 years	23				8			
< 5 years	26	$16.35	$21.05	$27.43	11			
Years In Position								
10+ years	48	$19.23	$25.85	$31.97	18			
5 - 9 years	32	$20.53	$26.84	$39.90	10			
< 5 years	73	$17.79	$23.08	$30.20	26	$37,800	$43,400	$49,500
Education (Highest Degree)								
doctoral degree	6				0			
master's degree	71	$20.19	$25.00	$32.96	27	$40,000	$48,000	$57,100
bachelor's degree	74	$18.19	$24.92	$32.78	26	$39,600	$46,900	$60,300
associate's degree	2				1			
Credentials Held								
RD	145	$19.28	$25.00	$33.67	51	$40,200	$47,900	$59,000
DTR	5				3			
state license	86	$19.23	$26.49	$31.30	28	$40,100	$46,600	$58,800
specialty certification(s)	11				2			
Employer								
self-employed	84	$22.10	$29.42	$39.26	11			
for-profit	23				16			
nonprofit (other than government)	19				11			
government	21				14			
Responsibilities								
director, manager or higher	53	$23.18	$28.85	$38.46	16			
supervise 1+ employees	42	$19.83	$27.14	$34.82	17			
supervise none	109	$18.11	$24.49	$32.50	37	$39,200	$46,800	$56,300
have budget responsibility	28	$20.29	$25.72	$31.20	18			
no budget responsibility	123	$18.99	$25.00	$33.33	35	$40,000	$46,700	$55,500

Note: Results not shown if fewer than 25 valid values.

Exhibit 7.35

Compensation: Consultant — Communications

Develops food and nutrition-related communications for consumer and/or professional audiences. May include writing speeches and presentations, developing nutrition education materials, programs, and nutrition content for Web sites, recipe development; and public speaking to consumer and health professional audiences.

| | HOURLY WAGE | | | | TOTAL CASH COMPENSATION (those employed full time, 1+ years) | | | |
	# answering	-- percentiles -- 25th	50th	75th	# answering	-- percentiles -- 25th	50th	75th
TOTAL	74	$20.11	$25.73	$39.15	28	$41,000	$52,500	$68,800
Years In Field								
20+ years	22				4			
10 - 19 years	29	$21.82	$28.85	$43.13	13			
5 - 9 years	15				7			
< 5 years	8				4			
Years In Position								
10+ years	18				8			
5 - 9 years	15				6			
< 5 years	41	$19.28	$25.00	$42.48	14			
Education (Highest Degree)								
doctoral degree	4				1			
master's degree	51	$20.15	$28.01	$42.79	19			
bachelor's degree	18				7			
associate's degree								
Credentials Held								
RD	70	$20.11	$26.37	$39.15	25	$42,600	$59,300	$69,500
DTR	4				3			
state license	35	$20.83	$25.64	$33.17	13			
specialty certification(s)	8				2			
Employer								
self-employed	38	$22.92	$31.88	$45.71	7			
for-profit	12				8			
nonprofit (other than government)	18				9			
government	6				4			
Responsibilities								
director, manager or higher	39	$21.63	$28.85	$38.46	14			
supervise 1+ employees	20				12			
supervise none	54	$20.11	$25.73	$39.15	16			
have budget responsibility	26	$19.65	$24.52	$39.54	9			
no budget responsibility	48	$20.96	$26.51	$40.28	19			

Note: Results not shown if fewer than 25 valid values.

Exhibit 7.36

Compensation: Sales Representative

Sells product and/or service. Establishes and maintains accounts with clients. Employed by pharmaceutical, medical/nutritional, food, or foodservice equipment or supplies company.

| | HOURLY WAGE | | | | TOTAL CASH COMPENSATION (those employed full time, 1+ years) | | | |
| | # | -- percentiles -- | | | # | -- percentiles -- | | |
	answering	25th	50th	75th	answering	25th	50th	75th
TOTAL	192	$22.26	$25.96	$32.80	164	$56,300	$70,000	$86,000
Years In Field								
20+ years	41	$25.31	$29.81	$36.06	36	$65,300	$76,500	$90,000
10 - 19 years	64	$24.04	$28.37	$34.88	56	$57,000	$76,000	$95,000
5 - 9 years	49	$22.76	$24.95	$29.09	42	$59,400	$65,800	$77,900
< 5 years	37	$18.15	$21.63	$24.76	30	$50,800	$55,100	$70,000
Years In Position								
10+ years	34	$30.29	$36.06	$39.78	32	$75,300	$89,500	$101,500
5 - 9 years	37	$24.04	$28.85	$33.89	33	$60,700	$77,000	$88,000
< 5 years	117	$21.59	$24.04	$26.85	99	$54,000	$63,000	$75,000
Education (Highest Degree)								
doctoral degree								
master's degree	90	$23.62	$26.88	$33.89	79	$60,000	$75,000	$95,000
bachelor's degree	97	$21.63	$25.11	$31.30	81	$54,600	$67,500	$81,000
associate's degree	4				3			
Credentials Held								
RD	184	$22.48	$26.44	$32.80	159	$58,000	$70,000	$86,000
DTR	5				4			
state license	67	$21.63	$25.48	$30.29	57	$55,100	$65,000	$88,500
specialty certification(s)	24				21			
Employer								
self-employed	3				1			
for-profit	186	$22.12	$26.20	$33.47	162	$56,600	$70,000	$86,000
nonprofit (other than government)	1				1			
government								
Responsibilities								
director, manager or higher	58	$24.04	$28.85	$36.06	52	$57,300	$75,000	$89,800
supervise 1+ employees	40	$24.28	$32.43	$39.42	38	$62,500	$82,200	$96,300
supervise none	152	$21.75	$25.30	$30.29	126	$54,800	$66,300	$80,800
have budget responsibility	112	$23.97	$26.44	$35.41	96	$62,100	$75,000	$94,800
no budget responsibility	79	$20.27	$25.00	$29.81	67	$48,000	$62,000	$78,300

Note: Results not shown if fewer than 25 valid values.

Exhibit 7.37

Compensation: Public Relations and/or Marketing Professional

Provides food and nutrition expertise in researching, designing, developing, implementing, and managing public relations and/or marketing programs for clients. May serve as a consultant or be employed by a PR agency, association, industry, or other organization/agency.

| | HOURLY WAGE | | | | TOTAL CASH COMPENSATION (those employed full time, 1+ years) | | | |
| | # answering | -- percentiles -- | | | # answering | -- percentiles -- | | |
		25th	50th	75th		25th	50th	75th
TOTAL	38	$23.56	$29.43	$36.54	29	$50,300	$62,500	$85,000
Years In Field								
20+ years	12				8			
10 - 19 years	12				10			
5 - 9 years	10				7			
< 5 years	4				4			
Years In Position								
10+ years	7				4			
5 - 9 years	10				8			
< 5 years	21				17			
Education (Highest Degree)								
doctoral degree								
master's degree	22				17			
bachelor's degree	16				12			
associate's degree								
Credentials Held								
RD	38	$23.56	$29.43	$36.54	29	$50,300	$62,500	$85,000
DTR								
state license	12				11			
specialty certification(s)	3				2			
Employer								
self-employed	7				2			
for-profit	18				16			
nonprofit (other than government)	12				10			
government								
Responsibilities								
director, manager or higher	27	$25.23	$33.65	$38.46	24			
supervise 1+ employees	20				19			
supervise none	18				10			
have budget responsibility	24				21			
no budget responsibility	14				8			

Note: Results not shown if fewer than 25 valid values.

Exhibit 7.38

Compensation: Corporate Dietitian

Provides nutrition and food information to customers and company employees; develops brochures, recipes, web site material, and promotional materials; organizes and attends special events, such as health fairs, trade shows, or media events. Employed by grocery retailer or other food-related company.

	HOURLY WAGE				TOTAL CASH COMPENSATION (those employed full time, 1+ years)			
	# answering	-- percentiles -- 25th	50th	75th	# answering	-- percentiles -- 25th	50th	75th
TOTAL	66	$17.79	$22.48	$28.85	44	$37,600	$48,500	$60,900
Years In Field								
20+ years	19				15			
10 - 19 years	15				10			
5 - 9 years	13				4			
< 5 years	19				15			
Years In Position								
10+ years	10				10			
5 - 9 years	11				5			
< 5 years	45	$16.30	$19.71	$24.15	29	$35,400	$41,000	$52,700
Education (Highest Degree)								
doctoral degree								
master's degree	34	$17.79	$23.78	$28.85	25	$38,400	$54,900	$62,000
bachelor's degree	29	$18.39	$21.63	$29.09	17			
associate's degree	3				2			
Credentials Held								
RD	62	$18.21	$22.82	$28.85	42	$38,400	$49,300	$61,600
DTR	4				2			
state license	29	$19.12	$24.13	$29.42	21			
specialty certification(s)	8				5			
Employer								
self-employed	4							
for-profit	49	$18.11	$22.44	$29.09	35	$38,000	$49,000	$65,000
nonprofit (other than government)	9				7			
government	3				1			
Responsibilities								
director, manager or higher	24				19			
supervise 1+ employees	33	$17.99	$21.63	$28.58	29	$38,700	$49,000	$61,400
supervise none	33	$16.83	$23.40	$29.67	15			
have budget responsibility	25	$19.47	$24.17	$31.25	23			
no budget responsibility	40	$16.27	$20.43	$27.40	20			

Note: Results not shown if fewer than 25 valid values.

Exhibit 7.39

Compensation: Research & Development Nutritionist

Develops recipes/products and marketing materials related to products; advises on Nutrition Facts panels and nutrient content/health claims; provides technical and written resources; designs research studies; analyzes and interprets nutrient research. May serve as a consultant or be employed by food, commodity, or medical/nutritional industry.

	HOURLY WAGE				TOTAL CASH COMPENSATION (those employed full time, 1+ years)			
	# answering	25th	50th	75th	# answering	25th	50th	75th
		-- percentiles --				-- percentiles --		
TOTAL	37	$21.88	$30.30	$37.93	32	$48,100	$64,400	$88,800
Years In Field								
20+ years	12				9			
10 - 19 years	12				12			
5 - 9 years	5				4			
< 5 years	8				7			
Years In Position								
10+ years	13				11			
5 - 9 years	8				8			
< 5 years	16				13			
Education (Highest Degree)								
doctoral degree	6				5			
master's degree	16				14			
bachelor's degree	14				12			
associate's degree	1				1			
Credentials Held								
RD	36	$22.36	$30.54	$38.44	31	$51,400	$65,900	$89,000
DTR	1				1			
state license	19				17			
specialty certification(s)	4				3			
Employer								
self-employed	3							
for-profit	30	$22.87	$31.01	$37.43	29	$49,200	$65,900	$88,500
nonprofit (other than government)	1				1			
government	3				2			
Responsibilities								
director, manager or higher	16				14			
supervise 1+ employees	14				13			
supervise none	23				19			
have budget responsibility	13				11			
no budget responsibility	24				21			

Note: Results not shown if fewer than 25 valid values.

Exhibit 7.40

Compensation: Manager of Nutrition Communications

Responsibilities may include managing nutrition education and nutrition marketing programs; developing, producing, and distributing nutrition communications; providing support and guidance to other areas of the organization. May include supervisory functions.

	HOURLY WAGE				TOTAL CASH COMPENSATION (those employed full time, 1+ years)			
	# answering	-- percentiles -- 25th	50th	75th	# answering	-- percentiles -- 25th	50th	75th
TOTAL	46	$20.49	$24.67	$33.95	35	$44,400	$52,300	$71,300
Years In Field								
20+ years	12				11			
10 - 19 years	19				13			
5 - 9 years	9				5			
< 5 years	6				6			
Years In Position								
10+ years	12				9			
5 - 9 years	11				9			
< 5 years	23				17			
Education (Highest Degree)								
doctoral degree								
master's degree	31	$20.44	$24.81	$35.58	25	$42,900	$56,900	$74,500
bachelor's degree	14				9			
associate's degree	1				1			
Credentials Held								
RD	44	$20.46	$24.67	$34.56	34	$44,000	$53,500	$72,000
DTR	1				1			
state license	19				15			
specialty certification(s)	8				7			
Employer								
self-employed								
for-profit	17				16			
nonprofit (other than government)	22				14			
government	7				5			
Responsibilities								
director, manager or higher	23				21			
supervise 1+ employees	23				18			
supervise none	23				17			
have budget responsibility	27	$20.51	$24.52	$35.58	22			
no budget responsibility	18				12			

Note: Results not shown if fewer than 25 valid values.

Exhibit 7.41

Compensation: Director of Nutrition

Responsibilities may include developing and executing the nutritional strategy of the company; tracking nutrition trends; identifying business opportunities; serving as company-wide resource on issues related to nutrition; representing the organization on nutritional and health committees and at meetings; managing a budget and staff.

	HOURLY WAGE				TOTAL CASH COMPENSATION (those employed full time, 1+ years)			
	# answering	-- percentiles -- 25th	50th	75th	# answering	-- percentiles -- 25th	50th	75th
TOTAL	99	$24.04	$29.23	$39.42	84	$53,900	$67,500	$85,900
Years In Field								
20+ years	54	$26.39	$34.62	$42.69	45	$58,100	$75,000	$108,400
10 - 19 years	26	$22.96	$25.99	$36.30	23			
5 - 9 years	13				11			
< 5 years	6				5			
Years In Position								
10+ years	49	$24.17	$33.65	$39.42	42	$53,100	$73,500	$87,800
5 - 9 years	19				13			
< 5 years	31	$23.08	$26.44	$34.86	29	$52,000	$67,000	$90,800
Education (Highest Degree)								
doctoral degree	13				12			
master's degree	50	$25.36	$30.02	$37.98	43	$54,300	$67,000	$82,500
bachelor's degree	34	$23.03	$25.57	$33.65	27	$50,800	$60,000	$76,000
associate's degree	2				2			
Credentials Held								
RD	97	$24.12	$29.74	$39.42	82	$54,200	$69,000	$87,200
DTR	2				2			
state license	50	$24.04	$28.66	$39.53	43	$53,900	$64,000	$82,500
specialty certification(s)	18				15			
Employer								
self-employed	5				3			
for-profit	41	$23.30	$33.65	$42.96	36	$56,800	$76,000	$106,300
nonprofit (other than government)	28	$25.58	$27.70	$38.87	25	$53,700	$60,000	$79,800
government	24				20			
Responsibilities								
director, manager or higher	85	$24.26	$30.29	$39.46	77	$54,500	$70,300	$88,900
supervise 1+ employees	90	$24.04	$29.49	$39.15	80	$54,000	$69,000	$85,900
supervise none	9				4			
have budget responsibility	86	$24.04	$29.04	$39.43	73	$53,700	$67,000	$88,900
no budget responsibility	12				10			

Note: Results not shown if fewer than 25 valid values.

Exhibit 7.42

Compensation: Instructor/Lecturer

Teaches undergraduate and/or graduate courses in food and nutrition related to area of expertise. May participate in research and service.

	HOURLY WAGE				TOTAL CASH COMPENSATION (those employed full time, 1+ years)			
	# answering	-- percentiles --			# answering	-- percentiles --		
		25th	50th	75th		25th	50th	75th
TOTAL	128	$19.24	$22.91	$30.04	26	$35,900	$42,600	$52,300
Years In Field								
20+ years	51	$16.78	$24.04	$30.00	7			
10 - 19 years	40	$20.92	$24.29	$32.81	4			
5 - 9 years	21				8			
< 5 years	16				7			
Years In Position								
10+ years	33	$19.98	$25.94	$32.57	6			
5 - 9 years	22				4			
< 5 years	72	$19.02	$21.76	$29.14	16			
Education (Highest Degree)								
doctoral degree	12				5			
master's degree	100	$19.23	$22.50	$29.49	17			
bachelor's degree	15				4			
associate's degree	1							
Credentials Held								
RD	121	$19.35	$23.08	$30.00	24			
DTR	7				2			
state license	61	$19.35	$22.00	$30.90	13			
specialty certification(s)	17				4			
Employer								
self-employed	3							
for-profit	19				1			
nonprofit (other than government)	55	$17.95	$22.12	$30.05	17			
government	46	$20.18	$23.38	$30.84	6			
Responsibilities								
director, manager or higher	5				4			
supervise 1+ employees	24				11			
supervise none	102	$19.23	$22.91	$30.00	15			
have budget responsibility	19				8			
no budget responsibility	108	$19.29	$22.61	$29.89	18			

Note: Results not shown if fewer than 25 valid values.

Exhibit 7.43

Compensation: Assistant Professor

Teaches undergraduate and/or graduate courses in food and nutrition related to area of expertise. Advises graduate and undergraduate students. Directs graduate student thesis/dissertation research. May conduct nutrition or food-related research.

| | HOURLY WAGE | | | | TOTAL CASH COMPENSATION (those employed full time, 1+ years) | | | |
| | # answering | -- percentiles -- | | | # answering | -- percentiles -- | | |
		25th	50th	75th		25th	50th	75th
TOTAL	56	$25.04	$29.75	$32.82	11			
Years In Field								
20+ years	21				4			
10 - 19 years	17				3			
5 - 9 years	15				4			
< 5 years	3							
Years In Position								
10+ years	12				1			
5 - 9 years	17				8			
< 5 years	27	$25.00	$27.08	$31.25	2			
Education (Highest Degree)								
doctoral degree	36	$26.75	$30.98	$33.33	8			
master's degree	20				3			
bachelor's degree								
associate's degree								
Credentials Held								
RD	55	$25.00	$29.69	$32.69	11			
DTR	1							
state license	26	$24.48	$26.39	$31.46	7			
specialty certification(s)	8				1			
Employer								
self-employed								
for-profit	8				1			
nonprofit (other than government)	23				3			
government	25	$25.61	$29.25	$33.33	7			
Responsibilities								
director, manager or higher	7				2			
supervise 1+ employees	28	$25.00	$31.25	$33.57	8			
supervise none	28	$25.98	$29.47	$31.38	3			
have budget responsibility	14				3			
no budget responsibility	42	$24.90	$29.69	$32.98	8			

Note: Results not shown if fewer than 25 valid values.

Exhibit 7.44

Compensation: Associate Professor

Teaches undergraduate and/or graduate courses in food and nutrition related to area of expertise. Advises graduate and undergraduate students. Directs graduate student thesis/dissertation research. Plans and conducts nutrition or food-related research.

	HOURLY WAGE				TOTAL CASH COMPENSATION (those employed full time, 1+ years)			
	# answering	-- percentiles --			# answering	-- percentiles --		
		25th	50th	75th		25th	50th	75th
TOTAL	58	$27.66	$31.25	$36.70	26	$55,500	$64,000	$72,300
Years In Field								
20+ years	41	$27.93	$31.28	$37.54	18			
10 - 19 years	15				7			
5 - 9 years	1				1			
< 5 years								
Years In Position								
10+ years	40	$27.49	$31.27	$37.95	18			
5 - 9 years	11				5			
< 5 years	7				3			
Education (Highest Degree)								
doctoral degree	44	$28.85	$32.57	$39.22	21			
master's degree	12				4			
bachelor's degree	2				1			
associate's degree								
Credentials Held								
RD	57	$27.57	$31.25	$36.96	25	$55,400	$64,000	$71,000
DTR	1				1			
state license	29	$27.93	$33.59	$40.10	13			
specialty certification(s)	10				3			
Employer								
self-employed								
for-profit	3							
nonprofit (other than government)	26	$23.98	$29.10	$36.70	11			
government	28	$29.33	$32.79	$38.24	14			
Responsibilities								
director, manager or higher	14				6			
supervise 1+ employees	39	$27.74	$31.72	$36.43	18			
supervise none	19				8			
have budget responsibility	26	$27.13	$31.27	$38.71	13			
no budget responsibility	31	$28.13	$30.77	$36.43	13			

Note: Results not shown if fewer than 25 valid values.

Exhibit 7.45

Compensation: Professor

Teaches undergraduate and/or graduate courses in food and nutrition related to area of expertise. Advises graduate and undergraduate students. Directs graduate student thesis/dissertation research. Establishes a nutrition or food-related research program.

	HOURLY WAGE				TOTAL CASH COMPENSATION (those employed full time, 1+ years)			
	# answering	-- percentiles --			# answering	-- percentiles --		
		25th	50th	75th		25th	50th	75th
TOTAL	43	$34.72	$40.48	$51.83	22			
Years In Field								
20+ years	34	$34.47	$44.60	$52.52	17			
10 - 19 years	9				5			
5 - 9 years								
< 5 years								
Years In Position								
10+ years	36	$34.76	$40.66	$51.77	20			
5 - 9 years	6				2			
< 5 years	1							
Education (Highest Degree)								
doctoral degree	38	$34.83	$40.66	$52.52	22			
master's degree	4							
bachelor's degree	1							
associate's degree								
Credentials Held								
RD	41	$34.80	$40.83	$51.88	21			
DTR								
state license	18				10			
specialty certification(s)	9				3			
Employer								
self-employed								
for-profit								
nonprofit (other than government)	26	$34.70	$43.81	$52.52	16			
government	17				6			
Responsibilities								
director, manager or higher	8				5			
supervise 1+ employees	34	$34.80	$45.45	$55.17	19			
supervise none	9				3			
have budget responsibility	28	$36.06	$46.23	$56.85	17			
no budget responsibility	14				5			

Note: Results not shown if fewer than 25 valid values.

Exhibit 7.46

Compensation: Administrator, Higher Education

Provides leadership in the development and evaluation of academic curricula, activities, and programs. Leads and facilitates strategic planning process for the college. Facilitates faculty appointment, promotion, tenure, and salary decisions. Requires doctorate degree.

	HOURLY WAGE				TOTAL CASH COMPENSATION (those employed full time, 1+ years)			
	# answering	-- percentiles -- 25th	50th	75th	# answering	-- percentiles -- 25th	50th	75th
TOTAL	27	$35.10	$43.85	$50.48	26	$76,800	$90,600	$107,200
Years In Field								
20+ years	23				22			
10 - 19 years	4				4			
5 - 9 years								
< 5 years								
Years In Position								
10+ years	18				18			
5 - 9 years	1				1			
< 5 years	8				7			
Education (Highest Degree)								
doctoral degree	21				20			
master's degree	6				6			
bachelor's degree								
associate's degree								
Credentials Held								
RD	27	$35.10	$43.85	$50.48	26	$76,800	$90,600	$107,200
DTR								
state license	10				10			
specialty certification(s)	4				4			
Employer								
self-employed								
for-profit	1				1			
nonprofit (other than government)	12				11			
government	14				14			
Responsibilities								
director, manager or higher	16				15			
supervise 1+ employees	25	$36.06	$43.85	$49.76	24			
supervise none	2				2			
have budget responsibility	22				21			
no budget responsibility	5				5			

Note: Results not shown if fewer than 25 valid values.

Exhibit 7.47

Compensation: Didactic Program Director

Assesses, plans, implements, and evaluates dietetics curriculum to meet and maintain CADE standards. Develops program information for potential and current students. Assures that educational competencies are included in appropriate courses. Recruits, advises, and counsels dietetic students. May teach undergraduate and graduate courses.

	HOURLY WAGE				TOTAL CASH COMPENSATION (those employed full time, 1+ years)			
	# answering	-- percentiles --			# answering	-- percentiles --		
		25th	50th	75th		25th	50th	75th
TOTAL	21				5			
Years In Field								
20+ years	16				4			
10 - 19 years	3				1			
5 - 9 years	2							
< 5 years								
Years In Position								
10+ years	13				3			
5 - 9 years	3							
< 5 years	5				2			
Education (Highest Degree)								
doctoral degree	4				1			
master's degree	15				2			
bachelor's degree	1				1			
associate's degree								
Credentials Held								
RD	20				4			
DTR	1				1			
state license	13				4			
specialty certification(s)	1							
Employer								
self-employed								
for-profit								
nonprofit (other than government)	12				1			
government	9				4			
Responsibilities								
director, manager or higher	16				3			
supervise 1+ employees	15				3			
supervise none	6				2			
have budget responsibility	10				1			
no budget responsibility	11				4			

Note: Results not shown if fewer than 25 valid values.

Exhibit 7.48

Compensation: Dietetic Internship Director

Assesses, plans, implements, and evaluates dietetic internship program to meet and maintain CADE standards. Coordinates and directs staff involved in the program. Plans and coordinates class and rotation schedules with staff and affiliation sites. May teach classes or perform other responsibilities separate from internship program.

	HOURLY WAGE				TOTAL CASH COMPENSATION (those employed full time, 1+ years)			
	# answering	25th	-- percentiles -- 50th	75th	# answering	25th	-- percentiles -- 50th	75th
TOTAL	52	$21.81	$24.51	$27.64	24			
Years In Field								
20+ years	28	$23.82	$25.00	$28.01	15			
10 - 19 years	17				4			
5 - 9 years	5				4			
< 5 years	1							
Years In Position								
10+ years	19				11			
5 - 9 years	10				3			
< 5 years	23				10			
Education (Highest Degree)								
doctoral degree	3				2			
master's degree	48	$21.64	$24.51	$26.89	22			
bachelor's degree	1							
associate's degree								
Credentials Held								
RD	52	$21.81	$24.51	$27.64	24			
DTR								
state license	33	$22.41	$24.52	$28.47	15			
specialty certification(s)	8				1			
Employer								
self-employed								
for-profit	2				1			
nonprofit (other than government)	22				9			
government	24				13			
Responsibilities								
director, manager or higher	36	$22.32	$24.45	$26.62	18			
supervise 1+ employees	28	$22.32	$24.51	$28.33	14			
supervise none	24				10			
have budget responsibility	31	$22.60	$24.51	$28.38	15			
no budget responsibility	21				9			

Note: Results not shown if fewer than 25 valid values.

Exhibit 7.49

Compensation: Research Dietitian

Collects data according to established protocols for research studies. Analyzes, interprets, and summarizes diet records and other research data. May supervise personnel and manage operational aspects of research program. May participate in grant and protocol writing and design.

	HOURLY WAGE				TOTAL CASH COMPENSATION (those employed full time, 1+ years)			
	# answering	-- percentiles -- 25th	50th	75th	# answering	-- percentiles -- 25th	50th	75th
TOTAL	175	$17.79	$21.15	$26.44	105	$38,700	$46,000	$55,700
Years In Field								
20+ years	49	$21.67	$25.96	$32.93	30	$49,000	$55,800	$74,800
10 - 19 years	51	$20.00	$23.08	$27.98	28	$42,600	$50,000	$57,800
5 - 9 years	38	$16.98	$19.23	$22.69	24			
< 5 years	37	$15.66	$17.79	$19.23	23			
Years In Position								
10+ years	36	$22.58	$25.84	$30.36	28	$47,600	$55,300	$69,400
5 - 9 years	36	$17.84	$22.15	$25.84	20			
< 5 years	103	$16.92	$19.42	$23.08	57	$37,000	$42,000	$51,000
Education (Highest Degree)								
doctoral degree	16				10			
master's degree	104	$19.23	$22.47	$27.94	64	$42,000	$49,800	$61,500
bachelor's degree	49	$16.80	$18.50	$23.04	28	$33,900	$41,700	$50,700
associate's degree	5				3			
Credentials Held								
RD	166	$18.23	$21.24	$26.79	101	$39,800	$46,300	$55,900
DTR	6				4			
state license	81	$18.06	$20.91	$24.39	50	$38,400	$45,000	$52,000
specialty certification(s)	23				14			
Employer								
self-employed	3							
for-profit	32	$17.85	$20.43	$25.36	20			
nonprofit (other than government)	92	$17.31	$21.15	$26.67	57	$38,400	$46,900	$59,000
government	45	$18.62	$22.19	$28.71	27	$38,800	$46,300	$62,000
Responsibilities								
director, manager or higher	31	$22.56	$27.40	$31.25	25	$46,100	$57,000	$67,400
supervise 1+ employees	102	$19.22	$22.58	$27.85	77	$39,800	$46,900	$59,000
supervise none	73	$16.25	$19.23	$23.04	28	$34,500	$42,500	$50,000
have budget responsibility	50	$20.19	$22.52	$28.89	39	$41,600	$46,800	$62,000
no budget responsibility	121	$17.31	$20.19	$25.36	64	$37,100	$45,000	$55,000

Note: Results not shown if fewer than 25 valid values.

8. Benefits

Notes

The tables in this section present survey results showing the proportion of dietetics practitioners offered each of a variety of benefits as part of their employment or self-employment.

Results are broken out in several different ways:

Registration status	RD DTR Not registered
Full-time status	Full-time Part-time
Employer status	Self-employed For-profit Nonprofit Government
Work setting (1)	Hospital Clinic or ambulatory care center Extended care facility Managed care organization, physician or other heathcare provider Community or public health program Government agency
Work setting (2)	School foodservice (K-12 or college/university) Private practice or consultation to individuals Consultation or contract services to organizations Contract food management company Food manufacturer, distributor, retailer College or university faculty
Size of organization (# employed at all locations)	1 (self-employed) 2 - 9 10 - 99 100 - 999 ≥1,000
Location (Census Division)	New England Middle Atlantic East North Central West North Central South Atlantic East South Central West South Central Mountain Pacific

Definitions of statistics reported and Census Divisions used to categorize employment location may be found in the *Appendix*.

Exhibit 8.1

Benefits By Registration Status

As of April 1, 2002, which of these benefits were offered as part of your employment/self-employment (whether you took advantage of them or not)?

	all practitioners	REGISTRATION STATUS		
		RD	DTR	not
base: practitioners (multiple answers)	10829 100%	9220 100%	1498 100%	111 100%
NET: paid time off	8987 83%	7515 82%	1382 92%	90 81%
paid vacation, personal time off	8730 81%	7300 79%	1345 90%	85 77%
paid holidays	8080 75%	6742 73%	1253 84%	85 77%
paid sick days	7967 74%	6688 73%	1198 80%	81 73%
NET: medical	8787 81%	7394 80%	1306 87%	87 78%
medical insurance, group plan, or savings account	8729 81%	7351 80%	1292 86%	86 77%
dental insurance or group plan	7907 73%	6655 72%	1173 78%	79 71%
prescription drug benefit	7349 68%	6224 68%	1060 71%	65 59%
vision insurance or group plan	5834 54%	4930 53%	856 57%	48 43%
NET: insurance	8034 74%	6770 73%	1198 80%	66 59%
life insurance	7536 70%	6351 69%	1127 75%	58 52%
disability insurance (long- and/or short-term)	6636 61%	5652 61%	934 62%	50 45%

Exhibit 8.1 (continued)

Benefits By Registration Status

As of April 1, 2002, which of these benefits were offered as part of your employment/self-employment (whether you took advantage of them or not)?

	all practitioners	REGISTRATION STATUS		
		RD	DTR	not
base: practitioners (multiple answers)	10829 100%	9220 100%	1498 100%	111 100%
NET: retirement, company stake	8255 76%	6996 76%	1185 79%	74 67%
defined contribution retirement plan (e.g., 401[k], SEP)	6850 63%	5877 64%	921 61%	52 47%
defined benefit retirement plan (pension)	4861 45%	4075 44%	735 49%	51 46%
stock options, ESOP	994 9%	859 9%	126 8%	9 8%
profit sharing	842 8%	730 8%	106 7%	6 5%
NET: professional development	6594 61%	5750 62%	806 54%	38 34%
funding for professional development (conferences, seminars, etc.)	6359 59%	5551 60%	772 52%	36 32%
professional society dues	2381 22%	2136 23%	235 16%	10 9%

Exhibit 8.1 (continued)

Benefits By Registration Status

As of April 1, 2002, which of these benefits were offered as part of your employment/self-employment (whether you took advantage of them or not)?

	all practitioners	REGISTRATION STATUS		
		RD	DTR	not
base: practitioners	10829	9220	1498	111
(multiple answers)	100%	100%	100%	100%
NET: family, wellness,	7846	6647	1133	66
workplace flexibility	72%	72%	76%	59%
college tuition assistance	4550	3792	729	29
	42%	41%	49%	26%
employee assistance or	4395	3733	639	23
wellness program	41%	40%	43%	21%
comp time or flex time	3803	3280	490	33
	35%	36%	33%	30%
fitness benefit (e.g., discounted health club member-ship, on-site facilities)	3177	2724	438	15
	29%	30%	29%	14%
extended and/or paid	2816	2407	392	17
parental leave	26%	26%	26%	15%
on-site child care	1328	1145	180	3
or allowance	12%	12%	12%	3%
telecommuting	740	692	42	6
	7%	8%	3%	5%
other	331	300	29	2
	3%	3%	2%	2%
indicated one or more	9636	8114	1426	96
	89%	88%	95%	86%
no benefits	1126	1050	64	12
	10%	11%	4%	11%
no answer	67	56	8	3
	1%	1%	1%	3%

Exhibit 8.2

Benefits By Full-Time Status

As of April 1, 2002, which of these benefits were offered as part of your employment/self-employment (whether you took advantage of them or not)?

	all practitioners	FULL-TIME?	
		yes	no
base: practitioners (multiple answers)	10829 100%	6967 100%	3153 100%
NET: paid time off	8987 83%	6754 97%	1904 60%
paid vacation, personal time off	8730 81%	6671 96%	1749 55%
paid holidays	8080 75%	6237 90%	1551 49%
paid sick days	7967 74%	6092 87%	1593 51%
NET: medical	8787 81%	6689 96%	1774 56%
medical insurance, group plan, or savings account	8729 81%	6652 95%	1758 56%
dental insurance or group plan	7907 73%	6130 88%	1501 48%
prescription drug benefit	7349 68%	5709 82%	1373 44%
vision insurance or group plan	5834 54%	4541 65%	1094 35%
NET: insurance	8034 74%	6180 89%	1571 50%
life insurance	7536 70%	5848 84%	1438 46%
disability insurance (long- and/or short-term)	6636 61%	5203 75%	1211 38%

Exhibit 8.2 (continued)

Benefits By Full-Time Status

As of April 1, 2002, which of these benefits were offered as part of your employment/self-employment (whether you took advantage of them or not)?

	all practitioners	FULL-TIME?	
		yes	no
base: practitioners (multiple answers)	10829 100%	6967 100%	3153 100%
NET: retirement, company stake	8255 76%	6192 89%	1768 56%
defined contribution retirement plan (e.g., 401[k], SEP)	6850 63%	5215 75%	1402 44%
defined benefit retirement plan (pension)	4861 45%	3665 53%	1029 33%
stock options, ESOP	994 9%	838 12%	119 4%
profit sharing	842 8%	656 9%	157 5%
NET: professional development	6594 61%	4873 70%	1474 47%
funding for professional development (conferences, seminars, etc.)	6359 59%	4688 67%	1438 46%
professional society dues	2381 22%	1879 27%	400 13%

Exhibit 8.2 (continued)

Benefits By Full-Time Status

As of April 1, 2002, which of these benefits were offered as part of your employment/self-employment (whether you took advantage of them or not)?

	all practitioners	FULL-TIME?	
		yes	no
base: practitioners (multiple answers)	10829 100%	6967 100%	3153 100%
NET: family, wellness, workplace flexibility	7846 72%	5828 84%	1735 55%
college tuition assistance	4550 42%	3529 51%	875 28%
employee assistance or wellness program	4395 41%	3324 48%	935 30%
comp time or flex time	3803 35%	2909 42%	776 25%
fitness benefit (e.g., discounted health club member-ship, on-site facilities)	3177 29%	2332 33%	746 24%
extended and/or paid parental leave	2816 26%	2193 31%	536 17%
on-site child care or allowance	1328 12%	979 14%	292 9%
telecommuting	740 7%	518 7%	171 5%
other	331 3%	237 3%	78 2%
indicated one or more	9636 89%	6859 98%	2345 74%
no benefits	1126 10%	100 1%	782 25%
no answer	67 1%	8 0%	26 1%

Exhibit 8.3

Benefits By Employer Status

As of April 1, 2002, which of these benefits were offered as part of your employment/self-employment (whether you took advantage of them or not)?

	all practitioners	EMPLOYER STATUS			
		self-employed	for-profit	non-profit	govt
base: practitioners (multiple answers)	10829 100%	1055 100%	3241 100%	4285 100%	2045 100%
NET: paid time off	8987 83%	100 9%	2852 88%	3954 92%	1934 95%
paid vacation, personal time off	8730 81%	90 9%	2804 87%	3859 90%	1840 90%
paid holidays	8080 75%	79 7%	2511 77%	3481 81%	1877 92%
paid sick days	7967 74%	60 6%	2401 74%	3483 81%	1896 93%
NET: medical	8787 81%	135 13%	2738 84%	3872 90%	1895 93%
medical insurance, group plan, or savings account	8729 81%	134 13%	2723 84%	3841 90%	1885 92%
dental insurance or group plan	7907 73%	51 5%	2514 78%	3573 83%	1637 80%
prescription drug benefit	7349 68%	69 7%	2310 71%	3271 76%	1575 77%
vision insurance or group plan	5834 54%	25 2%	1844 57%	2606 61%	1268 62%
NET: insurance	8034 74%	98 9%	2500 77%	3604 84%	1706 83%
life insurance	7536 70%	57 5%	2350 73%	3403 79%	1616 79%
disability insurance (long- and/or short-term)	6636 61%	75 7%	2174 67%	3065 72%	1223 60%

Exhibit 8.3 (continued)

Benefits By Employer Status

As of April 1, 2002, which of these benefits were offered as part of your employment/self-employment (whether you took advantage of them or not)?

	all practitioners	EMPLOYER STATUS			
		self-employed	for-profit	non-profit	govt
base: practitioners (multiple answers)	10829 100%	1055 100%	3241 100%	4285 100%	2045 100%
NET: retirement, company stake	8255 76%	130 12%	2552 79%	3651 85%	1797 88%
defined contribution retirement plan (e.g., 401[k], SEP)	6850 63%	99 9%	2336 72%	3053 71%	1262 62%
defined benefit retirement plan (pension)	4861 45%	29 3%	885 27%	2363 55%	1514 74%
stock options, ESOP	994 9%	13 1%	742 23%	176 4%	49 2%
profit sharing	842 8%	28 3%	556 17%	213 5%	28 1%
NET: professional development	6594 61%	228 22%	2060 64%	2861 67%	1349 66%
funding for professional development (conferences, seminars, etc.)	6359 59%	216 20%	1949 60%	2778 65%	1323 65%
professional society dues	2381 22%	142 13%	1030 32%	957 22%	220 11%

Exhibit 8.3 (continued)

Benefits By Employer Status

As of April 1, 2002, which of these benefits were offered as part of your employment/self-employment (whether you took advantage of them or not)?

	all practitioners	EMPLOYER STATUS			
		self-employed	for-profit	non-profit	govt
base: practitioners (multiple answers)	10829 100%	1055 100%	3241 100%	4285 100%	2045 100%
NET: family, wellness, workplace flexibility	7846 72%	154 15%	2329 72%	3540 83%	1697 83%
college tuition assistance	4550 42%	19 2%	1444 45%	2281 53%	731 36%
employee assistance or wellness program	4395 41%	15 1%	1110 34%	2199 51%	1014 50%
comp time or flex time	3803 35%	87 8%	968 30%	1540 36%	1135 56%
fitness benefit (e.g., discounted health club member-ship, on-site facilities)	3177 29%	41 4%	775 24%	1821 42%	489 24%
extended and/or paid parental leave	2816 26%	11 1%	805 25%	1292 30%	667 33%
on-site child care or allowance	1328 12%	14 1%	277 9%	816 19%	207 10%
telecommuting	740 7%	51 5%	250 8%	225 5%	202 10%
other	331 3%	39 4%	119 4%	98 2%	71 3%
indicated one or more	9636 89%	371 35%	3020 93%	4094 96%	1982 97%
no benefits	1126 10%	657 62%	200 6%	179 4%	57 3%
no answer	67 1%	27 3%	21 1%	12 0%	6 0%

Exhibit 8.4

Benefits By Work Setting (1)

As of April 1, 2002, which of these benefits were offered as part of your employment/self-employment (whether you took advantage of them or not)?

	all practitioners	hospital	clinic	extended care	managed care/ provider	public health program	govt agency
base: practitioners (multiple answers)	10829 100%	3613 100%	938 100%	1413 100%	167 100%	1002 100%	431 100%
NET: paid time off	8987 83%	3371 93%	840 90%	1167 83%	145 87%	916 91%	419 97%
paid vacation, personal time off	8730 81%	3330 92%	832 89%	1146 81%	144 86%	907 91%	411 95%
paid holidays	8080 75%	2904 80%	693 74%	1067 76%	141 84%	899 90%	413 96%
paid sick days	7967 74%	2941 81%	706 75%	986 70%	126 75%	884 88%	412 96%
NET: medical	8787 81%	3299 91%	814 87%	1108 78%	138 83%	880 88%	412 96%
medical insurance, group plan, or savings account	8729 81%	3276 91%	810 86%	1097 78%	138 83%	874 87%	410 95%
dental insurance or group plan	7907 73%	3076 85%	734 78%	982 69%	127 76%	803 80%	359 83%
prescription drug benefit	7349 68%	2826 78%	671 72%	879 62%	129 77%	733 73%	341 79%
vision insurance or group plan	5834 54%	2274 63%	546 58%	686 49%	110 66%	599 60%	294 68%
NET: insurance	8034 74%	3108 86%	759 81%	988 70%	130 78%	780 78%	360 84%
life insurance	7536 70%	2977 82%	707 75%	908 64%	122 73%	730 73%	338 78%
disability insurance (long- and/or short-term)	6636 61%	2651 73%	639 68%	755 53%	112 67%	600 60%	266 62%

Exhibit 8.4 (continued)

Benefits By Work Setting (1)

As of April 1, 2002, which of these benefits were offered as part of your employment/self-employment (whether you took advantage of them or not)?

	all practitioners	hospital	clinic	extended care	managed care/ provider	public health program	govt agency
base: practitioners (multiple answers)	10829 100%	3613 100%	938 100%	1413 100%	167 100%	1002 100%	431 100%
NET: retirement, company stake	8255 76%	3128 87%	794 85%	966 68%	133 80%	818 82%	388 90%
defined contribution retirement plan (e.g., 401[k], SEP)	6850 63%	2669 74%	707 75%	817 58%	115 69%	594 59%	274 64%
defined benefit retirement plan (pension)	4861 45%	1999 55%	394 42%	393 28%	76 46%	592 59%	340 79%
stock options, ESOP	994 9%	343 9%	107 11%	94 7%	11 7%	32 3%	7 2%
profit sharing	842 8%	237 7%	167 18%	68 5%	18 11%	24 2%	4 1%
NET: professional development	6594 61%	2359 65%	608 65%	793 56%	103 62%	666 66%	297 69%
funding for professional development (conferences, seminars, etc.)	6359 59%	2285 63%	599 64%	748 53%	100 60%	652 65%	291 68%
professional society dues	2381 22%	796 22%	139 15%	344 24%	27 16%	143 14%	49 11%

Exhibit 8.4 (continued)

Benefits By Work Setting (1)

As of April 1, 2002, which of these benefits were offered as part of your employment/self-employment (whether you took advantage of them or not)?

	all practitioners	hospital	clinic	extended care	managed care/ provider	public health program	govt agency
base: practitioners (multiple answers)	10829 100%	3613 100%	938 100%	1413 100%	167 100%	1002 100%	431 100%
NET: family, wellness, workplace flexibility	7846 72%	3040 84%	729 78%	917 65%	114 68%	773 77%	375 87%
college tuition assistance	4550 42%	2076 57%	448 48%	451 32%	75 45%	298 30%	137 32%
employee assistance or wellness program	4395 41%	1982 55%	412 44%	367 26%	72 43%	419 42%	241 56%
comp time or flex time	3803 35%	1242 34%	334 36%	487 34%	56 34%	547 55%	279 65%
fitness benefit (e.g., discounted health club membership, on-site facilities)	3177 29%	1690 47%	283 30%	212 15%	57 34%	176 18%	104 24%
extended and/or paid parental leave	2816 26%	1237 34%	265 28%	272 19%	39 23%	260 26%	143 33%
on-site child care or allowance	1328 12%	768 21%	120 13%	95 7%	14 8%	45 4%	50 12%
telecommuting	740 7%	117 3%	36 4%	35 2%	17 10%	63 6%	78 18%
other	331 3%	76 2%	25 3%	36 3%	4 2%	41 4%	12 3%
indicated one or more	9636 89%	3470 96%	875 93%	1239 88%	155 93%	944 94%	422 98%
no benefits	1126 10%	129 4%	58 6%	167 12%	12 7%	52 5%	7 2%
no answer	67 1%	14 0%	5 1%	7 0%	0 0%	6 1%	2 0%

Exhibit 8.5

Benefits By Work Setting (2)

As of April 1, 2002, which of these benefits were offered as part of your employment/self-employment (whether you took advantage of them or not)?

	all practitioners	school food-service	consult indivi-duals	consult organi-zations	food mgmt company	food mfr, dist, retailer	faculty
base: practitioners (multiple answers)	10829 100%	246 100%	427 100%	699 100%	210 100%	181 100%	491 100%
NET: paid time off	8987 83%	236 96%	84 20%	203 29%	199 95%	172 95%	394 80%
paid vacation, personal time off	8730 81%	200 81%	76 18%	198 28%	199 95%	170 94%	291 59%
paid holidays	8080 75%	207 84%	71 17%	182 26%	196 93%	170 94%	355 72%
paid sick days	7967 74%	233 95%	55 13%	156 22%	188 90%	144 80%	368 75%
NET: medical	8787 81%	239 97%	92 22%	222 32%	196 93%	165 91%	409 83%
medical insurance, group plan, or savings account	8729 81%	237 96%	92 22%	219 31%	196 93%	165 91%	408 83%
dental insurance or group plan	7907 73%	213 87%	49 11%	141 20%	193 92%	155 86%	352 72%
prescription drug benefit	7349 68%	198 80%	51 12%	152 22%	177 84%	152 84%	353 72%
vision insurance or group plan	5834 54%	159 65%	32 7%	91 13%	140 67%	131 72%	262 53%
NET: insurance	8034 74%	217 88%	69 16%	170 24%	196 93%	157 87%	360 73%
life insurance	7536 70%	210 85%	47 11%	147 21%	185 88%	144 80%	337 69%
disability insurance (long- and/or short-term)	6636 61%	162 66%	51 12%	137 20%	188 90%	146 81%	308 63%

Exhibit 8.5 (continued)

Benefits By Work Setting (2)

As of April 1, 2002, which of these benefits were offered as part of your employment/self-employment (whether you took advantage of them or not)?

	all practitioners	school food-service	consult indivi-duals	consult organi-zations	food mgmt company	food mfr, dist, retailer	faculty
base: practitioners	10829	246	427	699	210	181	491
(multiple answers)	100%	100%	100%	100%	100%	100%	100%
NET: retirement, company stake	8255	220	82	203	191	167	391
	76%	89%	19%	29%	91%	92%	80%
defined contribution retirement plan (e.g., 401[k], SEP)	6850	131	65	179	183	147	292
	63%	53%	15%	26%	87%	81%	59%
defined benefit retirement plan (pension)	4861	168	24	49	49	93	273
	45%	68%	6%	7%	23%	51%	56%
stock options, ESOP	994	10	5	33	101	60	5
	9%	4%	1%	5%	48%	33%	1%
profit sharing	842	2	16	35	65	53	4
	8%	1%	4%	5%	31%	29%	1%
NET: professional development	6594	185	114	221	176	147	293
	61%	75%	27%	32%	84%	81%	60%
funding for professional development (conferences, seminars, etc.)	6359	182	107	205	168	135	287
	59%	74%	25%	29%	80%	75%	58%
professional society dues	2381	67	75	128	151	127	65
	22%	27%	18%	18%	72%	70%	13%

Exhibit 8.5 (continued)

Benefits By Work Setting (2)

As of April 1, 2002, which of these benefits were offered as part of your employment/self-employment (whether you took advantage of them or not)?

	all practitioners	school food-service	consult indivi-duals	consult organi-zations	food mgmt company	food mfr, dist, retailer	faculty
base: practitioners	10829	246	427	699	210	181	491
(multiple answers)	100%	100%	100%	100%	100%	100%	100%
NET: family, wellness,	7846	173	88	189	171	152	379
workplace flexibility	72%	70%	21%	27%	81%	84%	77%
college tuition assistance	4550	75	18	60	134	95	267
	42%	30%	4%	9%	64%	52%	54%
employee assistance or	4395	84	22	43	99	84	200
wellness program	41%	34%	5%	6%	47%	46%	41%
comp time or flex time	3803	80	38	103	60	63	126
	35%	33%	9%	15%	29%	35%	26%
fitness benefit (e.g.,							
discounted health club member-	3177	41	38	37	36	61	174
ship, on-site facilities)	29%	17%	9%	5%	17%	34%	35%
extended and/or paid	2816	49	11	33	65	54	116
parental leave	26%	20%	3%	5%	31%	30%	24%
on-site child care	1328	12	13	14	17	16	64
or allowance	12%	5%	3%	2%	8%	9%	13%
telecommuting	740	7	21	54	27	49	90
	7%	3%	5%	8%	13%	27%	18%
other	331	12	13	32	5	21	10
	3%	5%	3%	5%	2%	12%	2%
indicated one or more	9636	243	193	352	203	177	449
	89%	99%	45%	50%	97%	98%	91%
no benefits	1126	2	221	337	6	3	39
	10%	1%	52%	48%	3%	2%	8%
no answer	67	1	13	10	1	1	3
	1%	0%	3%	1%	0%	1%	1%

ADA 2002 Dietetics Compensation & Benefits Survey

Exhibit 8.6

Benefits By Size of Organization

As of April 1, 2002, which of these benefits were offered as part of your employment/self-employment (whether you took advantage of them or not)?

	all practitioners	# OF EMPLOYEES (ALL LOCATIONS)				
		1	2 - 9	10 - 99	100 - 999	1000+
base: practitioners (multiple answers)	10829 100%	910 100%	616 100%	1541 100%	3207 100%	4207 100%
NET: paid time off	8987 83%	86 9%	458 74%	1310 85%	2929 91%	3998 95%
paid vacation, personal time off	8730 81%	79 9%	437 71%	1275 83%	2834 88%	3910 93%
paid holidays	8080 75%	71 8%	410 67%	1202 78%	2618 82%	3593 85%
paid sick days	7967 74%	62 7%	393 64%	1156 75%	2585 81%	3593 85%
NET: medical	8787 81%	118 13%	431 70%	1250 81%	2849 89%	3939 94%
medical insurance, group plan, or savings account	8729 81%	117 13%	426 69%	1240 80%	2824 88%	3924 93%
dental insurance or group plan	7907 73%	63 7%	360 58%	1061 69%	2543 79%	3701 88%
prescription drug benefit	7349 68%	64 7%	339 55%	994 65%	2348 73%	3445 82%
vision insurance or group plan	5834 54%	37 4%	254 41%	753 49%	1782 56%	2879 68%
NET: insurance	8034 74%	90 10%	375 61%	1069 69%	2586 81%	3738 89%
life insurance	7536 70%	64 7%	337 55%	972 63%	2426 76%	3580 85%
disability insurance (long- and/or short-term)	6636 61%	64 7%	291 47%	829 54%	2049 64%	3262 78%

Exhibit 8.6 (continued)

Benefits By Size of Organization

As of April 1, 2002, which of these benefits were offered as part of your employment/self-employment (whether you took advantage of them or not)?

	all practitioners	# OF EMPLOYEES (ALL LOCATIONS)				
		1	2 - 9	10 - 99	100 - 999	1000+
base: practitioners (multiple answers)	10829 100%	910 100%	616 100%	1541 100%	3207 100%	4207 100%
NET: retirement, company stake	8255 76%	109 12%	395 64%	1127 73%	2654 83%	3787 90%
defined contribution retirement plan (e.g., 401[k], SEP)	6850 63%	85 9%	318 52%	898 58%	2129 66%	3278 78%
defined benefit retirement plan (pension)	4861 45%	37 4%	218 35%	622 40%	1519 47%	2366 56%
stock options, ESOP	994 9%	6 1%	48 8%	105 7%	260 8%	559 13%
profit sharing	842 8%	13 1%	36 6%	139 9%	180 6%	459 11%
NET: professional development	6594 61%	183 20%	310 50%	898 58%	2125 66%	2944 70%
funding for professional development (conferences, seminars, etc.)	6359 59%	173 19%	299 49%	867 56%	2046 64%	2844 68%
professional society dues	2381 22%	105 12%	112 18%	301 20%	786 25%	1042 25%

Exhibit 8.6 (continued)

Benefits By Size of Organization

As of April 1, 2002, which of these benefits were offered as part of your employment/self-employment (whether you took advantage of them or not)?

	all practitioners	# OF EMPLOYEES (ALL LOCATIONS)				
		1	2 - 9	10 - 99	100 - 999	1000+
base: practitioners (multiple answers)	10829 100%	910 100%	616 100%	1541 100%	3207 100%	4207 100%
NET: family, wellness, workplace flexibility	7846 72%	139 15%	375 61%	1048 68%	2445 76%	3664 87%
college tuition assistance	4550 42%	22 2%	181 29%	455 30%	1301 41%	2504 60%
employee assistance or wellness program	4395 41%	18 2%	146 24%	445 29%	1321 41%	2371 56%
comp time or flex time	3803 35%	76 8%	174 28%	626 41%	1228 38%	1612 38%
fitness benefit (e.g., discounted health club membership, on-site facilities)	3177 29%	36 4%	125 20%	286 19%	894 28%	1784 42%
extended and/or paid parental leave	2816 26%	13 1%	99 16%	346 22%	803 25%	1503 36%
on-site child care or allowance	1328 12%	19 2%	46 7%	105 7%	294 9%	837 20%
telecommuting	740 7%	39 4%	39 6%	110 7%	196 6%	345 8%
other	331 3%	26 3%	18 3%	42 3%	94 3%	139 3%
indicated one or more	9636 89%	312 34%	520 84%	1407 91%	3058 95%	4098 97%
no benefits	1126 10%	571 63%	95 15%	119 8%	141 4%	102 2%
no answer	67 1%	27 3%	1 0%	15 1%	8 0%	7 0%

Exhibit 8.7

Benefits By Location (Census Division)

As of April 1, 2002, which of these benefits were offered as part of your employment/self-employment (whether you took advantage of them or not)?

	all practitioners	New England	Middle Atlantic	East North Central	West North Central	South Atlantic	East South Central	West South Central	Mountain	Pacific
base: practitioners (multiple answers)	10829 100%	740 100%	1692 100%	2136 100%	1008 100%	1754 100%	546 100%	879 100%	589 100%	1472 100%
NET: paid time off	8987 83%	574 78%	1411 83%	1869 88%	854 85%	1442 82%	465 85%	717 82%	464 79%	1180 80%
paid vacation, personal time off	8730 81%	563 76%	1380 82%	1806 85%	832 83%	1409 80%	454 83%	679 77%	447 76%	1149 78%
paid holidays	8080 75%	542 73%	1328 78%	1678 79%	760 75%	1267 72%	411 75%	606 69%	391 66%	1086 74%
paid sick days	7967 74%	528 71%	1300 77%	1623 76%	739 73%	1275 73%	404 74%	626 71%	396 67%	1065 72%
NET: medical	8787 81%	551 74%	1358 80%	1792 84%	835 83%	1417 81%	466 85%	722 82%	461 78%	1174 80%
medical insurance, group plan, or savings account	8729 81%	547 74%	1348 80%	1777 83%	832 83%	1403 80%	463 85%	720 82%	457 78%	1171 80%
dental insurance or group plan	7907 73%	501 68%	1219 72%	1624 76%	737 73%	1257 72%	401 73%	642 73%	415 70%	1104 75%
prescription drug benefit	7349 68%	432 58%	1168 69%	1538 72%	659 65%	1190 68%	391 72%	630 72%	374 63%	959 65%
vision insurance or group plan	5834 54%	285 39%	924 55%	1216 57%	492 49%	879 50%	278 51%	462 53%	322 55%	968 66%
NET: insurance	8034 74%	489 66%	1203 71%	1690 79%	772 77%	1310 75%	420 77%	671 76%	433 74%	1037 70%
life insurance	7536 70%	456 62%	1086 64%	1619 76%	744 74%	1229 70%	400 73%	651 74%	413 70%	929 63%
disability insurance (long- and/or short-term)	6636 61%	425 57%	983 58%	1407 66%	602 60%	1125 64%	317 58%	554 63%	355 60%	862 59%

Exhibit 8.7 (continued)

Benefits By Location (Census Division)

As of April 1, 2002, which of these benefits were offered as part of your employment/self-employment (whether you took advantage of them or not)?

	all practitioners	New England	Middle Atlantic	East North Central	West North Central	South Atlantic	East South Central	West South Central	Mountain	Pacific
base: practitioners (multiple answers)	10829 100%	740 100%	1692 100%	2136 100%	1008 100%	1754 100%	546 100%	879 100%	589 100%	1472 100%
NET: retirement, company stake	8255 76%	518 70%	1233 73%	1726 81%	796 79%	1327 76%	441 81%	669 76%	445 76%	1089 74%
defined contribution retirement plan (e.g., 401[k], SEP)	6850 63%	432 58%	966 57%	1420 66%	647 64%	1135 65%	380 70%	555 63%	377 64%	928 63%
defined benefit retirement plan (pension)	4861 45%	287 39%	782 46%	1077 50%	500 50%	748 43%	251 46%	362 41%	232 39%	615 42%
stock options, ESOP	994 9%	50 7%	131 8%	170 8%	78 8%	205 12%	79 14%	125 14%	53 9%	103 7%
profit sharing	842 8%	43 6%	103 6%	188 9%	77 8%	155 9%	50 9%	78 9%	51 9%	97 7%
NET: professional development	6594 61%	455 61%	948 56%	1396 65%	651 65%	1074 61%	346 63%	506 58%	350 59%	857 58%
funding for professional development (conferences, seminars, etc.)	6359 59%	439 59%	901 53%	1358 64%	635 63%	1030 59%	335 61%	480 55%	344 58%	826 56%
professional society dues	2381 22%	161 22%	389 23%	443 21%	210 21%	410 23%	149 27%	188 21%	125 21%	303 21%

Exhibit 8.7 (continued)

Benefits By Location (Census Division)

As of April 1, 2002, which of these benefits were offered as part of your employment/self-employment (whether you took advantage of them or not)?

	all practitioners	New England	Middle Atlantic	East North Central	West North Central	South Atlantic	East South Central	West South Central	Mountain	Pacific
base: practitioners (multiple answers)	10829 100%	740 100%	1692 100%	2136 100%	1008 100%	1754 100%	546 100%	879 100%	589 100%	1472 100%
NET: family, wellness, workplace flexibility	7846 72%	530 72%	1195 71%	1652 77%	770 76%	1267 72%	399 73%	601 68%	422 72%	1001 68%
college tuition assistance	4550 42%	348 47%	787 47%	1021 48%	425 42%	737 42%	225 41%	331 38%	237 40%	436 30%
employee assistance or wellness program	4395 41%	323 44%	578 34%	957 45%	484 48%	701 40%	178 33%	322 37%	241 41%	607 41%
comp time or flex time	3803 35%	221 30%	601 36%	870 41%	346 34%	619 35%	192 35%	281 32%	192 33%	477 32%
fitness benefit (e.g., discounted health club member-ship, on-site facilities)	3177 29%	250 34%	399 24%	689 32%	342 34%	484 28%	157 29%	262 30%	202 34%	386 26%
extended and/or paid parental leave	2816 26%	191 26%	402 24%	628 29%	260 26%	419 24%	140 26%	216 25%	146 25%	411 28%
on-site child care or allowance	1328 12%	98 13%	192 11%	306 14%	148 15%	221 13%	61 11%	88 10%	78 13%	135 9%
telecommuting	740 7%	47 6%	105 6%	124 6%	67 7%	118 7%	28 5%	60 7%	60 10%	131 9%
other	331 3%	24 3%	36 2%	66 3%	39 4%	44 3%	18 3%	31 4%	15 3%	56 4%
indicated one or more	9636 89%	624 84%	1494 88%	1987 93%	916 91%	1555 89%	499 91%	766 87%	510 87%	1274 87%
no benefits	1126 10%	112 15%	185 11%	135 6%	88 9%	190 11%	46 8%	109 12%	73 12%	186 13%
no answer	67 1%	4 1%	13 1%	14 1%	4 0%	9 1%	1 0%	4 0%	6 1%	12 1%

9. Practitioner Profile

Notes

The tables in this section present survey results profiling dietetics practitioners and their employment situations.

Included are tables describing employment status, demographic characteristics, professional qualifications, employment situations, and positions held. The first table is based on all 13,694 survey respondents; the remaining tables are based on the 10,829 respondents who were employed or self-employed in a dietetics-related position at the time of the survey. Note that respondents were instructed to respond with reference to their *primary* dietetics-related position if they were employed or self-employed in more than one.

Results are shown for all practitioners and are also split out by registration status: Registered Dietitians (RDs), Dietetics Technicians, Registered (DTRs), and those not registered.

The margins of error for percentages in each group are:

Segment	Base	Margin of Error
All practitioners	10,829	±0.9%
RDs	9,220	±0.9%
DTRs	1,498	±2.1%
Not registered	111	±9.0%

For definitions of statistics reported, Census Divisions used to categorize employment location, and standard position descriptions, refer to *Appendix*.

Exhibit 9.1

Employment Status

Are you currently employed or self-employed in a dietetics-related position?

	all practitioners	REGISTRATION STATUS		
		RD	DTR	not
base: all respondents	13694 100%	11607 100%	1892 100%	195 100%
yes	10829 79%	9220 79%	1498 79%	111 57%
no	2865 21%	2387 21%	394 21%	84 43%
no answer	0 0%	0 0%	0 0%	0 0%

Exhibit 9.2

Gender

Your gender?

	all practitioners	REGISTRATION STATUS		
		RD	DTR	not
base: practitioners	10829 100%	9220 100%	1498 100%	111 100%
female	10460 97%	8921 97%	1432 96%	107 96%
male	354 3%	285 3%	65 4%	4 4%
no answer	15 0%	14 0%	1 0%	0 0%

Exhibit 9.3

Age

Your age?

	all practitioners	REGISTRATION STATUS		
		RD	DTR	not
base: practitioners	10829	9220	1498	111
	100%	100%	100%	100%
65 or older	124	111	9	4
	1%	1%	1%	4%
60 - 64	350	294	53	3
	3%	3%	4%	3%
55 - 59	806	667	129	10
	7%	7%	9%	9%
50 - 54	1436	1210	209	17
	13%	13%	14%	15%
45 - 49	2044	1740	286	18
	19%	19%	19%	16%
40 - 44	1714	1400	308	6
	16%	15%	21%	5%
35 - 39	1295	1089	200	6
	12%	12%	13%	5%
30 - 34	1337	1187	142	8
	12%	13%	9%	7%
25 - 29	1436	1296	118	22
	13%	14%	8%	20%
under 25	249	196	37	16
	2%	2%	2%	14%
mean:	42.6	42.4	43.8	41.0
standard error:	0.1	0.1	0.2	1.2
median:	43	43	44	42
no answer	38	30	7	1
	0%	0%	0%	1%

Exhibit 9.4

Heritage

Are you Spanish, Hispanic, or Latino?

	all practitioners	REGISTRATION STATUS		
		RD	DTR	not
base: practitioners	10829 100%	9220 100%	1498 100%	111 100%
yes	282 3%	224 2%	42 3%	16 14%
no	10123 93%	8653 94%	1383 92%	87 78%
prefer not to disclose	217 2%	172 2%	42 3%	3 3%

Exhibit 9.5

Race

Your race?

	all practitioners	REGISTRATION STATUS		
		RD	DTR	not
base: practitioners	10829 100%	9220 100%	1498 100%	111 100%
White	9586 89%	8222 89%	1300 87%	64 58%
Asian, Native Hawaiian, or Pacific Islander	463 4%	412 4%	37 2%	14 13%
Black, African American, Negro	272 3%	190 2%	70 5%	12 11%
American Indian or Alaska Native	27 0%	23 0%	4 0%	0 0%
other	150 1%	110 1%	28 2%	12 11%
prefer not to disclose	272 3%	212 2%	53 4%	7 6%
no answer	59 1%	51 1%	6 0%	2 2%

Exhibit 9.6

Education

Highest level of education attained?

	all practitioners	REGISTRATION STATUS		
		RD	DTR	not
base: practitioners	10829	9220	1498	111
	100%	100%	100%	100%
doctoral degree	313	308	2	3
	3%	3%	0%	3%
master's degree	4213	4135	39	39
	39%	45%	3%	35%
bachelor's degree	5151	4745	347	59
	48%	51%	23%	53%
associate's degree	1124	7	1107	10
	10%	0%	74%	9%
other	21	19	2	0
	0%	0%	0%	0%
no answer	7	6	1	0
	0%	0%	0%	0%

Exhibit 9.7

Years in Field

Years of work experience in dietetics/nutrition? Exclude time taken off to return to school, raise a family, or work in other areas.

	all practitioners	REGISTRATION STATUS		
		RD	DTR	not
base: practitioners	10829	9220	1498	111
	100%	100%	100%	100%
30 years or more	835	770	51	14
	8%	8%	3%	13%
20 - 29 years	2895	2556	313	26
	27%	28%	21%	23%
15 - 19 years	1575	1337	231	7
	15%	15%	15%	6%
10 - 14 years	1590	1304	280	6
	15%	14%	19%	5%
5 - 9 years	1991	1611	371	9
	18%	17%	25%	8%
3 - 4 years	1029	866	148	15
	10%	9%	10%	14%
1 - 2 years	728	625	89	14
	7%	7%	6%	13%
less than 1 year	163	133	10	20
	2%	1%	1%	18%
mean:	15.3	15.6	13.7	13.0
standard error:	0.1	0.1	0.2	1.1
median:	15	15	12	9
no answer	23	18	5	0
	0%	0%	0%	0%

Exhibit 9.8

Registration Status

[from registration data]

	all practitioners	REGISTRATION STATUS		
		RD	DTR	not
base: practitioners	10829 100%	9220 100%	1498 100%	111 100%
RD	9216 85%	9216 100%	0 0%	0 0%
DTR	1498 14%	0 0%	1498 100%	0 0%
both	4 0%	4 0%	0 0%	0 0%
not registered	111 1%	0 0%	0 0%	111 100%
no answer	0 0%	0 0%	0 0%	0 0%

Exhibit 9.9

Year Registered

[from registration data]

	all practitioners	REGISTRATION STATUS		
		RD	DTR	not
base: practitioners	10829	9220	1498	111
	100%	100%	100%	100%
2000 or later	1304	1111	193	0
	12%	12%	13%	0%
1995 - 1999	2283	1816	467	0
	21%	20%	31%	0%
1990 - 1994	1744	1398	346	0
	16%	15%	23%	0%
1985 - 1989	1715	1223	492	0
	16%	13%	33%	0%
1980 - 1984	1377	1377	0	0
	13%	15%	0%	0%
1975 - 1979	1362	1362	0	0
	13%	15%	0%	0%
before 1975	933	933	0	0
	9%	10%	0%	0%
mean:	1988	1988	1993	
standard error:	0	0	0	
median:	1989	1988	1994	
not registered	111	0	0	111
	1%	0%	0%	100%
no answer	0	0	0	0
	0%	0%	0%	0%

Exhibit 9.10

Credentials Held

Dietetics/nutrition credentials held?

	all practitioners	REGISTRATION STATUS		
		RD	DTR	not
base: practitioners (multiple answers)	10829 100%	9220 100%	1498 100%	111 100%
RD (Registered Dietitian)	9253 85%	9220 100%	9 1%	24 22%
state license	4829 45%	4708 51%	87 6%	34 31%
specialty certifications (for example, CNSD, CDE, FADA, CSR, CSP, CHE, CDM, CFPP, CFE, CFM)	1604 15%	1510 16%	86 6%	8 7%
DTR (Dietetic Technician, Registered)	1522 14%	18 0%	1498 100%	6 5%
indicated one or more	10783 100%	9220 100%	1498 100%	65 59%
none of these	38 0%	0 0%	0 0%	38 34%
no answer	8 0%	0 0%	0 0%	8 7%

Exhibit 9.11

ADA Membership

[from membership data]

	all practitioners	REGISTRATION STATUS		
		RD	DTR	not
base: practitioners	10829	9220	1498	111
	100%	100%	100%	100%
yes	8775	7834	830	111
	81%	85%	55%	100%
no	2054	1386	668	0
	19%	15%	45%	0%
no answer	0	0	0	0
	0%	0%	0%	0%

Exhibit 9.12

Employer Status

Employer status for your primary position?

	all practitioners	REGISTRATION STATUS		
		RD	DTR	not
base: practitioners	10829	9220	1498	111
	100%	100%	100%	100%
nonprofit	4285	3535	714	36
(other than government)	40%	38%	48%	32%
for-profit	3241	2727	477	37
	30%	30%	32%	33%
government	2045	1782	233	30
	19%	19%	16%	27%
self-employed	1055	1012	37	6
	10%	11%	2%	5%
no answer	203	164	37	2
	2%	2%	2%	2%

Exhibit 9.13

Work Setting

Which ONE option best matches where you work in your primary position?

	all practitioners	REGISTRATION STATUS		
		RD	DTR	not
base: practitioners	10829 100%	9220 100%	1498 100%	111 100%
hospital	3613 33%	3031 33%	551 37%	31 28%
extended care facility	1413 13%	923 10%	473 32%	17 15%
community or public health program	1002 9%	849 9%	134 9%	19 17%
clinic or ambulatory care center	938 9%	907 10%	23 2%	8 7%
consultation or contract services to organizations	699 6%	679 7%	16 1%	4 4%
college or university faculty	491 5%	471 5%	17 1%	3 3%
government agency	431 4%	393 4%	32 2%	6 5%
private practice or consultation to individuals	427 4%	395 4%	22 1%	10 9%
school food service (K-12 or college/university)	246 2%	196 2%	49 3%	1 1%
contract food management company	210 2%	183 2%	25 2%	2 2%
food manufacturer, distributor, retailer	181 2%	164 2%	15 1%	2 2%
managed care organization, physician or other healthcare provider	167 2%	143 2%	24 2%	0 0%
home health care provider	86 1%	81 1%	5 0%	0 0%
other food service	46 0%	26 0%	19 1%	1 1%

Exhibit 9.13 (continued)

Work Setting

Which ONE option best matches where you work in your primary position?

	all practitioners	REGISTRATION STATUS		
		RD	DTR	not
base: practitioners	10829	9220	1498	111
	100%	100%	100%	100%
other:	857	763	87	7
	8%	8%	6%	6%
pharmaceutical or nutrition products company	85	85	0	0
	1%	1%	0%	0%
research unit or center	75	70	5	0
	1%	1%	0%	0%
dialysis unit	56	54	2	0
	1%	1%	0%	0%
other	641	554	80	7
	6%	6%	5%	6%
no answer	22	16	6	0
	0%	0%	0%	0%

Exhibit 9.14

Employment Location

What is the zip code of your primary work location?

	all practitioners	REGISTRATION STATUS		
		RD	DTR	not
CENSUS DIVISION				
base: practitioners	10829 100%	9220 100%	1498 100%	111 100%
New England	740 7%	614 7%	123 8%	3 3%
Middle Atlantic	1692 16%	1305 14%	348 23%	39 35%
East North Central	2136 20%	1697 18%	428 29%	11 10%
West North Central	1008 9%	875 9%	130 9%	3 3%
South Atlantic	1754 16%	1534 17%	194 13%	26 23%
East South Central	546 5%	511 6%	28 2%	7 6%
West South Central	879 8%	819 9%	56 4%	4 4%
Mountain	589 5%	544 6%	40 3%	5 5%
Pacific	1472 14%	1308 14%	151 10%	13 12%
no answer	13 0%	13 0%	0 0%	0 0%

Exhibit 9.15

Size of Organization

Including you, how many people are employed by your organization?

	all practitioners	REGISTRATION STATUS		
		RD	DTR	not
base: practitioners	10829	9220	1498	111
	100%	100%	100%	100%
1,000 or more	4207	3709	467	31
	39%	40%	31%	28%
500 - 999	1110	948	154	8
	10%	10%	10%	7%
250 - 499	1009	819	179	11
	9%	9%	12%	10%
100 - 249	1088	815	255	18
	10%	9%	17%	16%
50 - 99	505	405	93	7
	5%	4%	6%	6%
25 - 49	507	421	80	6
	5%	5%	5%	5%
10 - 24	529	427	94	8
	5%	5%	6%	7%
5 - 9	354	293	52	9
	3%	3%	3%	8%
2 - 4	262	215	43	4
	2%	2%	3%	4%
1 (yourself only)	910	870	33	7
	8%	9%	2%	6%
mean:	541.6	552.0	486.9	414.8
standard error:	4.2	4.6	10.8	40.0
median:	534	603	354	214
no answer	348	298	48	2
	3%	3%	3%	2%

Exhibit 9.16

Primary Practice Area

Which ONE option best matches the practice area where you spend the most time in this position?

	all practitioners	REGISTRATION STATUS		
		RD	DTR	not
base: practitioners	10829	9220	1498	111
	100%	100%	100%	100%
clinical nutrition	5780	4860	870	50
	53%	53%	58%	45%
food and nutrition management	1663	1250	388	25
	15%	14%	26%	23%
community	1417	1259	142	16
	13%	14%	9%	14%
consultation and business	914	881	24	9
	8%	10%	2%	8%
education and research	872	828	38	6
	8%	9%	3%	5%
no answer	183	142	36	5
	2%	2%	2%	5%

Exhibit 9.17

Primary Position

Please carefully review the enclosed list of Position Descriptions. Which ONE description most closely matches your primary position (even if the job title differs)?

	all practitioners	REGISTRATION STATUS		
		RD	DTR	not
base: practitioners	10829	9220	1498	111
	100%	100%	100%	100%
SUBTOTAL: CLINICAL NUTRITION — ACUTE CARE/INPATIENT	3213	2576	609	28
	30%	28%	41%	25%
Dietetic Technician, Clinical	601	18	578	5
	6%	0%	39%	5%
Clinical Dietitian	1553	1508	25	20
	14%	16%	2%	18%
Clinical Dietitian, Specialist — Bariatrics	14	14	0	0
	0%	0%	0%	0%
Clinical Dietitian, Specialist — Cardiac	67	65	1	1
	1%	1%	0%	1%
Clinical Dietitian, Specialist — Developmental disorders	25	24	0	1
	0%	0%	0%	1%
Clinical Dietitian, Specialist — Diabetes	142	142	0	0
	1%	2%	0%	0%
Clinical Dietitian, Specialist — Eating disorders	20	19	1	0
	0%	0%	0%	0%
Clinical Dietitian, Specialist — HIV/AIDS	19	19	0	0
	0%	0%	0%	0%
Clinical Dietitian, Specialist — Oncology	73	73	0	0
	1%	1%	0%	0%
Clinical Dietitian, Specialist — Psychiatric	37	35	2	0
	0%	0%	0%	0%
Clinical Dietitian, Specialist — Renal	233	232	1	0
	2%	3%	0%	0%
Clinical Dietitian, Specialist — Substance abuse	3	3	0	0
	0%	0%	0%	0%
Clinical Dietitian, Specialist — Surgery	25	24	0	1
	0%	0%	0%	1%

Exhibit 9.17 (continued)

Primary Position

Please carefully review the enclosed list of Position Descriptions. Which ONE description most closely matches your primary position (even if the job title differs)?

	all practitioners	REGISTRATION STATUS		
		RD	DTR	not
base: practitioners	10829	9220	1498	111
	100%	100%	100%	100%
Clinical Dietitian, Specialist — Transplant	17	17	0	0
	0%	0%	0%	0%
Pediatric/Neonatal Dietitian	173	173	0	0
	2%	2%	0%	0%
Nutrition Support Dietitian	211	210	1	0
	2%	2%	0%	0%
SUBTOTAL: CLINICAL NUTRITION — AMBULATORY CARE	1288	1273	8	7
	12%	14%	1%	6%
Outpatient Dietitian, General	364	362	1	1
	3%	4%	0%	1%
Outpatient Dietitian, Specialist — Allergy	2	2	0	0
	0%	0%	0%	0%
Outpatient Dietitian, Specialist — Cardiac Rehabilitation	41	41	0	0
	0%	0%	0%	0%
Outpatient Dietitian, Specialist — Diabetes	363	361	0	2
	3%	4%	0%	2%
Outpatient Dietitian, Specialist — Eating disorders	29	28	1	0
	0%	0%	0%	0%
Outpatient Dietitian, Specialist — Oncology	32	32	0	0
	0%	0%	0%	0%
Outpatient Dietitian, Specialist — Pediatrics	61	60	0	1
	1%	1%	0%	1%
Outpatient Dietitian, Specialist — Renal	250	247	2	1
	2%	3%	0%	1%
Outpatient Dietitian, Specialist — Weight Management	67	63	2	2
	1%	1%	0%	2%
Home Care Dietitian	79	77	2	0
	1%	1%	0%	0%

Exhibit 9.17 (continued)

Primary Position

Please carefully review the enclosed list of Position Descriptions. Which ONE description most closely matches your primary position (even if the job title differs)?

	all practitioners	REGISTRATION STATUS		
		RD	DTR	not
base: practitioners	10829 100%	9220 100%	1498 100%	111 100%
SUBTOTAL: CLINICAL NUTRITION — LONG TERM CARE	1383 13%	1071 12%	299 20%	13 12%
Clinical Dietitian, Long Term Care	1133 10%	1063 12%	58 4%	12 11%
Dietetic Technician, Long Term Care	250 2%	8 0%	241 16%	1 1%
SUBTOTAL: EDUCATION AND RESEARCH	614 6%	592 6%	17 1%	5 5%
Instructor/Lecturer	150 1%	142 2%	8 1%	0 0%
Assistant Professor	64 1%	63 1%	1 0%	0 0%
Associate Professor	67 1%	66 1%	1 0%	0 0%
Professor	45 0%	43 0%	0 0%	2 2%
Administrator, Higher Education	30 0%	30 0%	0 0%	0 0%
Didactic Program Director	23 0%	22 0%	1 0%	0 0%
Dietetic Internship Director	55 1%	55 1%	0 0%	0 0%
Research Dietitian	180 2%	171 2%	6 0%	3 3%

Exhibit 9.17 (continued)

Primary Position

Please carefully review the enclosed list of Position Descriptions. Which ONE description most closely matches your primary position (even if the job title differs)?

	all practitioners	REGISTRATION STATUS		
		RD	DTR	not
base: practitioners	10829 100%	9220 100%	1498 100%	111 100%
SUBTOTAL: COMMUNITY	1188 11%	1024 11%	143 10%	21 19%
WIC Nutritionist	605 6%	493 5%	101 7%	11 10%
Public Health Nutritionist	324 3%	313 3%	8 1%	3 3%
Cooperative Extension Educator/Specialist	95 1%	77 1%	17 1%	1 1%
School/Child Care Nutritionist	73 1%	61 1%	10 1%	2 2%
Corrections Dietitian	18 0%	17 0%	0 0%	1 1%
Nutrition Coordinator for Head Start Program	46 0%	39 0%	5 0%	2 2%
Nutritionist for Food Bank or Assistance Program	27 0%	24 0%	2 0%	1 1%
SUBTOTAL: FOOD AND NUTRITION MANAGEMENT	1557 14%	1231 13%	305 20%	21 19%
Executive-level Professional	201 2%	184 2%	13 1%	4 4%
Director of Food and Nutrition Services	589 5%	485 5%	95 6%	9 8%
Clinical Nutrition Manager	349 3%	345 4%	3 0%	1 1%
Assistant Foodservice Director	138 1%	109 1%	25 2%	4 4%
School Foodservice Director	118 1%	93 1%	24 2%	1 1%

Exhibit 9.17 (continued)

Primary Position

Please carefully review the enclosed list of Position Descriptions. Which ONE description most closely matches your primary position (even if the job title differs)?

	all practitioners	REGISTRATION STATUS		
		RD	DTR	not
base: practitioners	10829 100%	9220 100%	1498 100%	111 100%
Dietetic Technician, Foodservice Management	162 1%	15 0%	145 10%	2 2%
SUBTOTAL: CONSULTATION AND BUSINESS	1096 10%	1051 11%	35 2%	10 9%
Private Practice Dietitian — Patient/Client Nutrition Care	331 3%	316 3%	12 1%	3 3%
Consultant — Community and/or Corporate Programs	172 2%	164 2%	5 0%	3 3%
Consultant — Communications	84 1%	79 1%	5 0%	0 0%
Sales Representative	204 2%	196 2%	5 0%	3 3%
Public Relations and/or Marketing Professional	42 0%	42 0%	0 0%	0 0%
Corporate Dietitian	72 1%	68 1%	4 0%	0 0%
Research & Development Nutritionist	42 0%	41 0%	1 0%	0 0%
Manager of Nutrition Communications	48 0%	46 0%	1 0%	1 1%
Director of Nutrition	101 1%	99 1%	2 0%	0 0%
OTHER	327 3%	278 3%	46 3%	3 3%
no answer	163 2%	124 1%	36 2%	3 3%

Exhibit 9.18

Responsibility Level

What is this position's responsibility level?

	all practitioners	REGISTRATION STATUS		
		RD	DTR	not
base: practitioners	10829 100%	9220 100%	1498 100%	111 100%
owner or partner	609 6%	578 6%	24 2%	7 6%
executive	161 1%	150 2%	6 0%	5 5%
director or manager	2354 22%	2021 22%	313 21%	20 18%
supervisor or coordinator	2272 21%	1888 20%	356 24%	28 25%
other	5294 49%	4460 48%	787 53%	47 42%
no answer	139 1%	123 1%	12 1%	4 4%

Exhibit 9.19

Number Supervised

In this position, how many employees do you directly or indirectly supervise (if any)?

	all practitioners	REGISTRATION STATUS		
		RD	DTR	not
base: practitioners	10829	9220	1498	111
	100%	100%	100%	100%
supervise one or more:	5232	4405	762	65
	48%	48%	51%	59%
100 or more	237	212	23	2
	2%	2%	2%	2%
50 - 99	343	300	37	6
	3%	3%	2%	5%
25 - 49	628	497	120	11
	6%	5%	8%	10%
10 - 24	1288	950	320	18
	12%	10%	21%	16%
5 - 9	926	802	114	10
	9%	9%	8%	9%
3 - 4	725	647	72	6
	7%	7%	5%	5%
1 - 2	1085	997	76	12
	10%	11%	5%	11%
mean:	20.1	19.9	21.1	22.6
standard error:	0.4	0.4	0.8	3.1
median:	8	8	15	13
none	5558	4786	726	46
	51%	52%	48%	41%
no answer	39	29	10	0
	0%	0%	1%	0%

Exhibit 9.20

Budget Responsibility

In this position, approximately what is the size of the budget you manage (if applicable)?

	all practitioners	REGISTRATION STATUS		
		RD	DTR	not
base: practitioners	10829	9220	1498	111
	100%	100%	100%	100%
manage a budget:	2880	2491	358	31
	27%	27%	24%	28%
$1 million or more	736	678	50	8
	7%	7%	3%	7%
$500,000 - $999,999	360	313	43	4
	3%	3%	3%	4%
$250,000 - $499,999	396	331	60	5
	4%	4%	4%	5%
$100,000 - $249,999	559	447	106	6
	5%	5%	7%	5%
$50,000 - $99,999	267	227	38	2
	2%	2%	3%	2%
$25,000 - $49,999	207	171	33	3
	2%	2%	2%	3%
less than $25,000	355	324	28	3
	3%	4%	2%	3%
mean:	$446,000	$459,000	$357,000	$459,000
standard error:	$7,000	$8,000	$18,000	$71,000
median:	$283,000	$308,000	$214,000	$312,000
does not apply	7685	6539	1070	76
	71%	71%	71%	68%
no answer	264	190	70	4
	2%	2%	5%	4%

Exhibit 9.21

Years In Position

How many years have you worked in this primary dietetics-related position?

	all practitioners	REGISTRATION STATUS		
		RD	DTR	not
base: practitioners	10829	9220	1498	111
	100%	100%	100%	100%
30 years or more	181	158	17	6
	2%	2%	1%	5%
20 - 29 years	951	792	143	16
	9%	9%	10%	14%
15 - 19 years	877	743	128	6
	8%	8%	9%	5%
10 - 14 years	1492	1250	229	13
	14%	14%	15%	12%
5 - 9 years	2219	1832	382	5
	20%	20%	26%	5%
3 - 4 years	1683	1411	257	15
	16%	15%	17%	14%
1 - 2 years	3046	2704	310	32
	28%	29%	21%	29%
less than 1 year	352	304	31	17
	3%	3%	2%	15%
mean:	7.8	7.8	8.3	8.5
standard error:	0.1	0.1	0.2	0.9
median:	5	5	6	3
no answer	28	26	1	1
	0%	0%	0%	1%

Exhibit 9.22

Position Pay Base: Hours Per Week

As of April 1, 2002, how many HOURS PER WEEK and WEEKS PER YEAR was this position's pay based on?

	all practitioners	REGISTRATION STATUS		
		RD	DTR	not
HOURS PER WEEK				
base: answering practitioners	10120	8621	1397	102
	100%	100%	100%	100%
40 hours or more	6448	5430	952	66
	64%	63%	68%	65%
35 - 39 hours	806	651	131	24
	8%	8%	9%	24%
30 - 34 hours	698	589	106	3
	7%	7%	8%	3%
20 - 29 hours	1258	1103	151	4
	12%	13%	11%	4%
10 - 19 hours	569	523	44	2
	6%	6%	3%	2%
less than 10 hours	341	325	13	3
	3%	4%	1%	3%
mean:	34.6	34.4	36.2	37.0
standard error:	0.1	0.1	0.2	0.8
median:	40	40	40	40

Exhibit 9.23

Position Pay Base: Weeks Per Year

As of April 1, 2002, how many HOURS PER WEEK and WEEKS PER YEAR was this position's pay based on?

	all practitioners	REGISTRATION STATUS		
		RD	DTR	not
WEEKS PER YEAR				
base: answering practitioners	10120 100%	8621 100%	1397 100%	102 100%
52 weeks	8916 88%	7535 87%	1298 93%	83 81%
48 - 51 weeks	617 6%	560 6%	46 3%	11 11%
44 - 47 weeks	128 1%	117 1%	9 1%	2 2%
40 - 43 weeks	197 2%	172 2%	23 2%	2 2%
36 - 39 weeks	113 1%	103 1%	8 1%	2 2%
32 - 25 weeks	33 0%	30 0%	2 0%	1 1%
26 - 31 weeks	57 1%	46 1%	10 1%	1 1%
less than 26 weeks	59 1%	58 1%	1 0%	0 0%
mean:	51.0	50.9	51.4	50.6
standard error:	0.0	0.0	0.1	0.4
median:	52	52	52	52

Exhibit 9.24

Position Pay Base: Hours Per Year

As of April 1, 2002, how many HOURS PER WEEK and WEEKS PER YEAR was this position's pay based on?

	all practitioners	REGISTRATION STATUS		
		RD	DTR	not
HOURS PER YEAR				
base: answering practitioners	10120	8621	1397	102
	100%	100%	100%	100%
2080 hours	5996	5042	898	56
(40 hours x 52 weeks)	59%	58%	64%	55%
1820 - 2079 hours	972	793	152	27
(≥35 hours x 52 weeks)	10%	9%	11%	26%
1560 - 1819 hours	776	655	116	5
(≥30 hours x 52 weeks)	8%	8%	8%	5%
1040 - 1559 hours	1338	1165	165	8
(≥20 hours x 52 weeks)	13%	14%	12%	8%
520 - 1039 hours	618	565	50	3
(≥10 hours x 52 weeks)	6%	7%	4%	3%
less than 520 hours	420	401	16	3
(<10 hours x 52 weeks)	4%	5%	1%	3%
mean:	1760	1744	1853	1858
standard error:	5	6	11	40
median:	2080	2080	2080	2080

Exhibit 9.25

Position Pay Base: Incidence of Full-Time Employment

As of April 1, 2002, how many HOURS PER WEEK and WEEKS PER YEAR was this position's pay based on?

	all practitioners	REGISTRATION STATUS		
		RD	DTR	not
FULL-TIME EMPLOYMENT ≥35 hours per week ≥48 weeks per year				
base: answering practitioners	10120 100%	8621 100%	1397 100%	102 100%
employed full-time	6967 69%	5833 68%	1050 75%	84 82%
employed less than full-time	3153 31%	2788 32%	347 25%	18 18%

10. Appendix

Methodological Notes

Sample Composition and Disposition The survey sample of 30,000 was selected by Readex, Inc., the ADA's survey contractor, in systematic stratified fashion from the population of all domestic Active and Active-Eligible ADA members (N =55,084) plus all domestic nonmembers (N = 18,654) maintaining current registration as a Registered Dietitian (RD) or Dietetic Technician, Registered (DTR). Because of their relatively small numbers, the sample was stratified to overrepresent DTRs.

A total of 13,694 responses was received, for a 46% response rate overall. The response rate was highest among RDs, lowest among those not registered. Although a 46% response rate represents a strong showing for a mail survey of this type, possible effects of nonresponse bias need to be considered in interpreting results.

Most data tables are based on the 10,829 practitioners currently employed in a dietetics-related position. The margin of error (maximum sampling error for percentages at the 95% confidence level) is ±0.9% overall.

The table below details population, sample, and response by registration status and by ADA membership:

| | Registration | | | |
	RD	DTR	None	TOTAL
POPULATION				
ADA members	50,727	2,375	1,982	55,084
Not ADA members	16,206	2,448		18,654
TOTAL	66,933	4,823	1,982	73,738
SAMPLE				
ADA members	18,532	2,375	724	21,631
Not ADA members	5,921	2,448		8,369
TOTAL	24,453	4,823	724	30,000
RESPONSE				
ADA members	9,312	1,011	195	10,518
Not ADA members	2,295	881		3,176
TOTAL	11,607	1,892	195	13,694
Response rate	47%	39%	27%	46%
Employed practitioners	9,220	1,498	111	10,829
Margin of error	±0.9%	±2.1%	±9.0%	±0.9%

Instrument Design A groundbreaking feature of the 2002 ADA Dietetics Compensation & Benefits Survey was the measurement of salary data not only in the context of registration (RD, DTR) or various practice areas, but also in terms of the specific jobs (including nontraditional jobs) held by dietetics professionals.

The core set of dietetics job titles plus brief position descriptions was developed through an extended process involving ADA member input and expert judgment. The resulting set of 58 positions proved to cover 95% of responding practitioners' situations.

The questionnaire was developed jointly by the ADA's Salary Survey Workgroup and Readex, Inc., the survey contractor. A panel of ADA members critiqued the draft instrument, adding valuable perspective.

Mailing Series Production of survey materials, addressing, and mailing were all handled by Readex.

On July 10, 2002, Readex mailed survey kits to all 30,000 sample members. Each kit consisted of a cover letter on ADA letterhead, signed by the association's Chief Executive Officer (with a *2002 Survey* order form on the back); a Position Descriptions list; the questionnaire; and a Business Reply envelope addressed to Readex, all in an outgoing ADA envelope.

On July 31, Readex mailed followup survey kits to the 22,689 sample members who had not responded by that time. The follow-up survey kits were similar to the initial survey kits, with the exception of an updated covering letter.

The survey was closed for tabulation on August 26, 2002. Data entry, verification, cleaning and tabulation were handled by Readex.

Geographic Definitions

In various tables, survey results are broken out by employment location: Census Division, state, or metropolitan area.

The metropolitan areas reported are those defined by the Office of Management and Budget (OMB) for purposes of collecting, tabulating, and publishing federal data. They are used extensively by the US Census Bureau and represent large population nucleii, together with adjacent communities having a high degree of social and economic integration with that core. Metropolitan areas comprise one or more entire counties, except in New England, where cities and towns are the basic geographic units. For more information, see www.census.gov/population/www/estimates/metrodef.html.

The Census Divisions reported are also standards employed by the US Census Bureau. The 50 states are divided into 9 geographic divisions with similar aggregate characteristics. The map below shows how the 9 Divisions are defined:

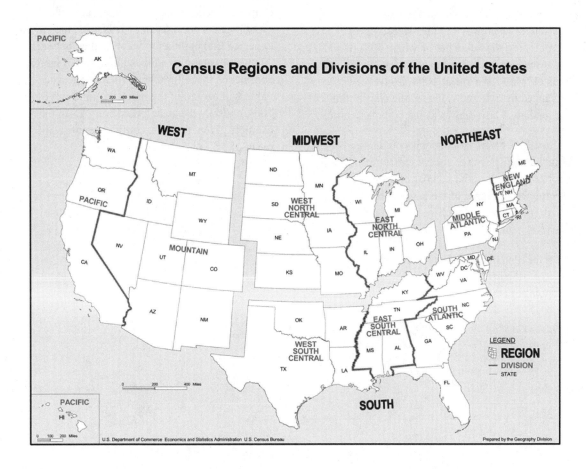

Statistical Glossary

base The divisor in calculations of percentages.

margin of error The maximum sampling error for percentages at the 95% confidence level. If the margin of error is ±1%, then the expected true population value will be within ±1% of the survey's estimated value 95 times out of 100.

mean The arithmetic average, calculated by summing all responses and dividing by the number of responses. The mean is sometimes strongly influenced by extreme values in the distribution.

median The median is calculated by rank ordering all responses and then selecting (or interpolating) the value below which 50% of all responses lie. It is often thought of as the "typical" value of a variable and is not influenced by extreme values in the distribution. The median is also known as the 50th percentile.

net In tables where respondents could select more than one answer, a net is sometimes reported, indicating the number of respondents selecting one or more of the answers being netted. Each respondent is counted at most once in a net.

percentile Percentiles are calculated by rank ordering all responses and then selecting (or interpolating) the value below which x% of all responses lie: 10% of all answers lie below the 10th percentile, 25% below the 25th percentile, and so on.

regression model Regression models, such as those upon which this report's Salary Calculation Worksheets are based, are developed with multivariate statistical procedures that result in a linear equation relating a number of predictor variables to the dependent variable of interest (in this report, hourly wage). Given satisfaction of key assumptions and moderate predictive power, they provide an unbiased estimator of the dependent variable within known margins of error.

standard error The "margin of error" for estimated means based on survey data. If the standard error for a mean of 2.5 is 0.5, then the expected true population value will be between 2.0 and 3.0 about two times in three. To increase confidence to the 95% level (that is, the true value will be within the range 95 times out of 100), multiply the standard error by 2. In the example given, the 95% confidence interval for a mean of 2.5 is 1.5 to 3.5.

Title Index: Compensation By Position

Practice Area

Position Title

Title Index: Compensation By Position (continued)

Position Title

Position Descriptions

POSITION DESCRIPTIONS

Clinical Nutrition — Acute Care/Inpatient

A01: Dietetic Technician, Clinical

Conducts nutrition screening and routine assessments. Coordinates menu selections with diet order. Develops and implements nutrition care plans for assigned patients. Provides individualized or group nutrition education. Monitors quality and accuracy of food served to patients.

A02: Clinical Dietitian

Performs comprehensive nutrition assessments. Develops and implements nutrition care plans. Provides medical nutrition therapy and nutrition education. May coordinate and supervise activities of DTRs and students.

Clinical Dietitian, Specialist

In addition to the duties described for the Clinical Dietitian, provides medical nutrition therapy for inpatients in a specialty area (devotes more than 50% of time to this specialty):

A03:	Bariatrics	A09:	Oncology
A04:	Cardiac	A10:	Psychiatric
A05:	Developmental disorders	A11:	Renal
A06:	Diabetes	A12:	Substance abuse
A07:	Eating disorders	A13:	Surgery
A08:	HIV/AIDS	A14:	Transplant

A15: Pediatric/Neonatal Dietitian

Performs nutrition assessments and consults for pediatric patients. Develops, implements, and monitors effectiveness of age-appropriate nutrition care plans. Provides nutrition counseling and education.

A16: Nutrition Support Dietitian

Obtains and interprets nutrition assessment data to triage critically ill patients. Develops and implements individualized nutrition support care plans. Monitors nutritional status of patients receiving nutrition support.

Clinical Nutrition — Ambulatory Care

B01: Outpatient Dietitian, General

Assesses the nutritional health of outpatients. Develops and implements individualized care plans. Provides nutrition education to individuals and groups.

Outpatient Dietitian, Specialist

In addition to the duties described for the Outpatient Dietitian, provides medical nutrition therapy for outpatients in a specialty area (devotes more than 50% of time to this specialty):

B02:	Allergy	B06:	Oncology
B03:	Cardiac Rehabilitation	B07:	Pediatrics
B04:	Diabetes	B08:	Renal
B05:	Eating disorders	B09:	Weight Management

B10: Home Care Dietitian

Provides nutrition services to patients in a home care setting. Consults with case managers and physicians on screening and assessment of patients. Monitors and evaluates nutrition care of high-risk patients.

Clinical Nutrition — Long Term Care

C01: Clinical Dietitian, Long Term Care

Develops and implements nutrition care plans for residents. Documents progress and recommendations. Provides nutrition education for residents, families, and staff. May consult with foodservice staff on food preparation, service, and delivery. May provide services as a consultant to more than one facility or be employed by single facility.

C02: Dietetic Technician, Long Term Care

Performs nutrition screening and routine assessments, and provides basic nutrition care. Monitors resident satisfaction and tolerance of meals. May monitor food production and meal service.

Education and Research

D01: Instructor/Lecturer

Teaches undergraduate and/or graduate courses in food and nutrition related to area of expertise. May participate in research and service.

D02: Assistant Professor

Teaches undergraduate and/or graduate courses in food and nutrition related to area of expertise. Advises graduate and undergraduate students. Directs graduate student thesis/dissertation research. May conduct nutrition or food-related research.

D03: Associate Professor

Teaches undergraduate and/or graduate courses in food and nutrition related to area of expertise. Advises graduate and undergraduate students. Directs graduate student thesis/dissertation research. Plans and conducts nutrition or food-related research.

D04: Professor

Teaches undergraduate and/or graduate courses in food and nutrition related to area of expertise. Advises graduate and undergraduate students. Directs graduate student thesis/dissertation research. Establishes a nutrition or food-related research program.

D05: Administrator, Higher Education

Provides leadership in the development and evaluation of academic curricula, activities, and programs. Leads and facilitates strategic planning process for the college. Facilitates faculty appointment, promotion, tenure, and salary decisions. Requires doctorate degree.

D06: Didactic Program Director

Assesses, plans, implements, and evaluates dietetics curriculum to meet and maintain CADE standards. Develops program information for potential and current students. Assures that educational competencies are included in appropriate courses. Recruits, advises, and counsels dietetic students. May teach undergraduate and graduate courses.

D07: Dietetic Internship Director

Assesses, plans, implements, and evaluates dietetic internship program to meet and maintain CADE standards. Coordinates and directs staff involved in the program. Plans and coordinates class and rotation schedules with staff and affiliation sites. May teach classes or perform other responsibilities separate from internship program.

D08: Research Dietitian

Collects data according to established protocols for research studies. Analyzes, interprets, and summarizes diet records and other research data. May supervise personnel and manage operational aspects of research program. May participate in grant and protocol writing and design.

E01: WIC Nutritionist

Contributes to the development, implementation, and evaluation of the nutrition education component of the WIC program. Provides nutrition therapy and education for WIC clients. Offers technical assistance to WIC staff. May provide supervision and training for WIC staff.

E02: Public Health Nutritionist

Contributes to the planning, development, coordination, and evaluation of public health nutrition programs. Assesses community nutritional needs and develops related standards and services. May counsel patients on normal and therapeutic nutrition. May provide supervision and training for public health department staff.

E03: Cooperative Extension Educator/Specialist

Develops, implements, and evaluates educational programs and materials addressing family and community needs. Conducts family and consumer educational programs. Responds to general, family, consumer, food safety, food, and nutrition questions. May involve a faculty appointment to an affiliated university.

E04: School/Child Care Nutritionist

Plans, develops, and implements school and childcare nutrition programs and resources. Monitors and evaluates menus and foodservice programs. Consults with parents and school leaders on nutritional needs of high-risk children.

E05: Corrections Dietitian

Plans, directs, and coordinates food and nutrition services for inmates. Monitors and evaluates menus for normal and therapeutic diets. Provides diet instructions for inmates. May supervise and train foodservice personnel.

E06: Nutrition Coordinator for Head Start Program

Designs and implements nutrition programs that meet the nutritional needs and feeding requirements of each child. Provides counseling to parents of children at nutritional risk. Plans menus and special meals. May supervise foodservice operations.

E07: Nutritionist for Food Bank or Assistance Program

Performs client nutrition assessments and follow-ups, and refers and advocates for clients to other service providers. Conducts nutrition education workshops for clients, staff, and community groups. Monitors and evaluates nutritional content and quality assurance of food products. May supervise and train staff.

Food and Nutrition Management

F01: Executive-level Professional

Plans, controls, and directs services/operations for multiple departments, product lines, or facilities. Accountable for quality of services, financial results, and achievement of organizational objectives.

F02: Director of Food and Nutrition Services

Plans, coordinates, and evaluates the personnel and activities of the food and nutrition services department. Directs food and equipment purchasing. Manages budget and human resource needs of staff. Develops and implements department policies and procedures.

F03: Clinical Nutrition Manager

Plans, organizes, and manages clinical nutrition services. Recruits, trains, supervises, and evaluates clinical nutrition staff. Develops and implements policies and procedures. Manages human resources and budget. May also perform duties of a patient services manager.

F04: Assistant Foodservice Director

Manages daily operations of foodservice department. Directs and supervises the preparation and service of food. Recruits, trains, supervises, and evaluates foodservice staff. Assists in managing budget.

F05: School Foodservice Director

Develops, implements, and maintains the foodservice program in a school setting. Directs and monitors food procurement and storage, and food production, assembly, and service to students. Plans menus to meet required nutritional standards and student acceptance.

F06: Dietetic Technician, Foodservice Management

Oversees meal production, service, and delivery. Manages employee orientation, training, performance evaluations, scheduling, and assignment of tasks. Assures compliance with standards, policies, and procedures.

Consultation and Business

G01: Private Practice Dietitian— Patient/Client Nutrition Care

Provides medical nutrition therapy or wellness, fitness, or sports nutrition counseling for individuals or groups in a private practice setting or healthcare provider's office.

G02: Consultant — Community and/or Corporate Programs

Provides food and nutrition consultation services for community-based programs, such as meal programs, day care centers, or group homes. Develops and implements wellness events and programs for communities and/or corporations.

G03: Consultant — Communications

Develops food and nutrition-related communications for consumer and/or professional audiences. May include writing speeches and presentations, developing nutrition education materials, programs, and nutrition content for Web sites, recipe development; and public speaking to consumer and health professional audiences.

G04: Sales Representative

Sells product and/or service. Establishes and maintains accounts with clients. Employed by pharmaceutical, medical/nutritional, food, or foodservice equipment or supplies company.

G05: Public Relations and/or Marketing Professional

Provides food and nutrition expertise in researching, designing, developing, implementing, and managing public relations and/or marketing programs for clients. May serve as a consultant or be employed by a PR agency, association, industry, or other organization/agency.

G06: Corporate Dietitian

Provides nutrition and food information to customers and company employees; develops brochures, recipes, web site material, and promotional materials; organizes and attends special events, such as health fairs, trade shows, or media events. Employed by grocery retailer or other food-related company.

G07: Research & Development Nutritionist

Develops recipes/products and marketing materials related to products; advises on Nutrition Facts panels and nutrient content/health claims; provides technical and written resources; designs research studies; analyzes and interprets nutrient research. May serve as a consultant or be employed by food, commodity, or medical/nutritional industry.

G08: Manager of Nutrition Communications

Responsibilities may include managing nutrition education and nutrition marketing programs; developing, producing, and distributing nutrition communications; providing support and guidance to other areas of the organization. May include supervisory functions.

G09: Director of Nutrition

Responsibilities may include developing and executing the nutritional strategy of the company; tracking nutrition trends; identifying business opportunities; serving as company-wide resource on issues related to nutrition; representing the organization on nutritional and health committees and at meetings; managing a budget and staff.

Other

000: Other Position Not Listed

Questionnaire

AMERICAN DIETETIC ASSOCIATION 2002 Dietetics Compensation & Benefits Survey

About your current employment

1. Are you currently employed or self-employed in a dietetics-related position?

A dietetics-related position is considered to be any position that requires or makes use of your education, training, and/or experience in dietetics or nutrition, including situations outside of "traditional" dietetics practice. See enclosed Position Descriptions for some examples.

☐ yes, I am currently employed or self-employed in a dietetics-related position

☐ no ... this survey will not apply to you. Please ✓ no and return the form in the postage-paid envelope provided. Thank you!

> *Please answer the remaining questions for what you consider to be your **primary** dietetics-related position (if you are employed/self-employed in more than one).*

2. Employer status for your primary position?

☐ self-employed ☐ non-profit (other than government)
☐ for-profit ☐ government

3. Which *one* option best matches where you work in your primary position? *(please ✓ the one best option)*

☐ private practice or consultation to individuals
☐ consultation or contract services to organizations
☐ hospital
☐ clinic or ambulatory care center
☐ extended care facility

☐ home health care provider
☐ managed care organization, physician or other healthcare provider
☐ community or public health program
☐ government agency

☐ school food service (K-12 or college/university)
☐ other food service
☐ contract food management company
☐ food manufacturer, distributor, retailer
☐ college or university faculty

☐ other: _____

4. What is the zip code of your primary work location?

__ __ __ __ __

5. Including you, how many people are employed by your organization? By your practice, if self-employed.

Please count all types of positions at ALL locations, full- and part-time.

☐ 1 (yourself only) ☐ 50 - 99
☐ 2 - 4 ☐ 100 - 249
☐ 5 - 9 ☐ 250 - 499
☐ 10 - 24 ☐ 500 - 999
☐ 25 - 49 ☐ 1,000 or more

About your current position

1. How many years have you worked in this primary dietetics-related position?

#_____ years in this position

2. Which *one* option best matches the practice area where you spend the most time in this position?
(please ✓ the one best option)

☐ clinical nutrition
☐ food and nutrition management
☐ community
☐ consultation and business
☐ education and research

3. What is your current job title?

_____

4. Please carefully review the enclosed list of Position Descriptions. Which *one* description most closely matches your primary position (even if the job title differs)?
(fill in the 3-character code found next to the position title)

__ __ __

> *Response to this item is critical for data analysis — please don't skip!*

5. What is this position's responsibility level?

☐ owner or partner ☐ supervisor or coordinator
☐ executive ☐ other
☐ director or manager

6. In this position, how many employees do you directly or indirectly supervise (if any)?

☐ none ☐ 10 - 24
☐ 1 - 2 ☐ 25 - 49
☐ 3 - 4 ☐ 50 - 99
☐ 5 - 9 ☐ 100 or more

7. In this position, approximately what is the size of the budget you manage (if applicable)?

☐ does not apply ☐ $100,000 - $249,999
☐ less than $25,000 ☐ $250,000 - $499,999
☐ $25,000 - $49,999 ☐ $500,000 - $999,999
☐ $50,000 - $99,999 ☐ $1 million or more

8. As of April 1, 2002, how many *hours per week* and *weeks per year* was this position's pay based on? If self-employed, how many hours and weeks typically worked?

Please fill in a number for both — for example, 40 hours per week and 52 weeks per year for a typical full-time year-round position. Do not count overtime, on-call hours, etc.

#_____ hours per week #_____ weeks per year

PLEASE TURN OVER >>>

9a. As of April 1, 2002, what was the annual salary or wage for this position?

Please include only the regular salary/wage paid for your primary position. **Exclude** earnings from other work, overtime pay, on-call pay, commissions, bonuses, incentive pay, profit sharing, retirement benefits received, and the monetary value of any other benefits.

If you are self-employed, please fill in the amount you paid yourself as salary or draw (if any), **not** total practice revenues or lump-sum profit distributions.

$ ___ ___ ___ , ___ ___ ___ per year

9b. In the 12 months prior to April 1, 2002, approximately what was the total value of all OTHER cash compensation received for this position (if any)?

Please estimate if exact figures are not readily available. **Exclude** regular salary/wage and earnings from other work. **Include** overtime pay, on-call pay, commissions, bonuses, incentive pay, profit sharing or distributions, and cash retirement benefits received. Exclude the monetary value of any other benefits.

$ ___ ___ ___ , ___ ___ ___ other cash compensation

☐ NO OTHER CASH COMPENSATION BEYOND SALARY/WAGE

10. As of April 1, 2002, which of these benefits were offered as part of your employment/self-employment (whether you took advantage of them or not)?

If self-employed, please include only those benefits explicitly funded in your practice's budget.

☐ paid holidays
☐ paid sick days
☐ paid vacation, personal time off
☐ comp time or flex time
☐ telecommuting

☐ medical insurance, group plan, or savings account
☐ prescription drug benefit
☐ dental insurance or group plan
☐ vision insurance or group plan
☐ life insurance

☐ disability insurance (long- and/or short-term)
☐ on-site child care or allowance
☐ extended and/or paid parental leave
☐ employee assistance or wellness program
☐ fitness benefit (e.g., discounted health club membership, on-site facilities)

☐ defined benefit retirement plan (pension)
☐ defined contribution retirement plan (e.g., 401(k), SEP)
☐ profit sharing
☐ stock options, ESOP
☐ professional society dues

☐ funding for professional development (conferences, seminars, etc.)
☐ college tuition assistance

☐ other: _____

☐ NO BENEFITS

About you

1. Your gender?

☐ female   ☐ male

2. Your age?

☐ under 25   ☐ 45 - 49
☐ 25 - 29   ☐ 50 - 54
☐ 30 - 34   ☐ 55 - 59
☐ 35 - 39   ☐ 60 - 64
☐ 40 - 44   ☐ 65 or over

3a. Are you Spanish, Hispanic, or Latino?

☐ yes   ☐ no   ☐ PREFER NOT TO DISCLOSE

3b. Your race?

☐ White
☐ Black, African American, Negro
☐ American Indian or Alaska Native
☐ Asian, Native Hawaiian, or Pacific Islander
☐ other
☐ PREFER NOT TO DISCLOSE

4. Highest level of education attained?

☐ doctoral degree
☐ masters degree
☐ bachelors degree
☐ associates degree
☐ other

5. Years of work experience in dietetics/nutrition?

Exclude time taken off to return to school, raise a family, or work in other areas.

☐ less than 1 year   ☐ 10 - 14 years
☐ 1 - 2 years   ☐ 15 - 19 years
☐ 3 - 4 years   ☐ 20 - 29 years
☐ 5 - 9 years   ☐ 30 years or more

6. Dietetics/nutrition credentials held?
(please ✓ all that apply)

☐ RD (Registered Dietitian)
☐ DTR (Dietetic Technician, Registered)
☐ state license
☐ specialty certifications (for example, CNSD, CDE, FADA, CSR, CSP, CHE, CDM, CFPP, CFE, CFM)
☐ NONE OF THESE

7. To what e-mail address shall we send the Executive Summary of these survey results?

_____

THANK YOU!

(Please check that you've answered all questions on both pages, then return your survey using the postage-paid reply envelope provided.)

2002 ADA Compensation and Benefits Survey
RESPONSE FORM

In an effort to provide you with compensation and benefits information that meets your evolving needs as a dietetics professional, please take a moment to provide your comments and suggestions. By answering the following questions, you will help us continue to be your premier source for compensation and benefits information for the dietetics professional.

Did you find the survey results easy to understand?   Yes ___ No ___
If no, what changes would make them easier to understand?

Did this survey provide the information you need regarding compensation issues?   Yes ___ No ___
If no, what additional information could we provide?

Did this survey provide the information you need regarding benefits issues?   Yes ___ No ___
If no, what additional information could we provide?

Any additional comments or suggestions?

(Optional) Name _____

Organization _____

Return by mail or fax to:
Vice President, Member Services
American Dietetic Association
216 W. Jackson Blvd., Chicago, IL 60606
Fax: 312-899-4812